SPORTS AND ATHLETICS PREPARATION, PERFORMANCE,
AND PSYCHOLOGY

SPORTS MEDICINE AND TRAINING TOOLS

SPORTS AND ATHLETICS PREPARATION, PERFORMANCE, AND PSYCHOLOGY

Additional books in this series can be found on Nova's website under the Series tab.

Additional E-books in this series can be found on Nova's website under the E-books tab.

SPORTS AND ATHLETICS PREPARATION, PERFORMANCE,
AND PSYCHOLOGY

SPORTS MEDICINE AND TRAINING TOOLS

BRENDA D. CARMICHAEL
AND
ALAN B. MITCHELL
EDITORS

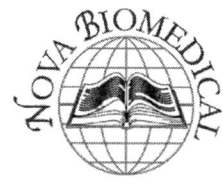

Nova Science Publishers, Inc.
New York

Copyright © 2011 by Nova Science Publishers, Inc.

All rights reserved. No part of this book may be reproduced, stored in a retrieval system or transmitted in any form or by any means: electronic, electrostatic, magnetic, tape, mechanical photocopying, recording or otherwise without the written permission of the Publisher.

For permission to use material from this book please contact us:
Telephone 631-231-7269; Fax 631-231-8175
Web Site: http://www.novapublishers.com

NOTICE TO THE READER

The Publisher has taken reasonable care in the preparation of this book, but makes no expressed or implied warranty of any kind and assumes no responsibility for any errors or omissions. No liability is assumed for incidental or consequential damages in connection with or arising out of information contained in this book. The Publisher shall not be liable for any special, consequential, or exemplary damages resulting, in whole or in part, from the readers' use of, or reliance upon, this material. Any parts of this book based on government reports are so indicated and copyright is claimed for those parts to the extent applicable to compilations of such works.

Independent verification should be sought for any data, advice or recommendations contained in this book. In addition, no responsibility is assumed by the publisher for any injury and/or damage to persons or property arising from any methods, products, instructions, ideas or otherwise contained in this publication.

This publication is designed to provide accurate and authoritative information with regard to the subject matter covered herein. It is sold with the clear understanding that the Publisher is not engaged in rendering legal or any other professional services. If legal or any other expert assistance is required, the services of a competent person should be sought. FROM A DECLARATION OF PARTICIPANTS JOINTLY ADOPTED BY A COMMITTEE OF THE AMERICAN BAR ASSOCIATION AND A COMMITTEE OF PUBLISHERS.

Additional color graphics may be available in the e-book version of this book.

LIBRARY OF CONGRESS CATALOGING-IN-PUBLICATION DATA

Sports medicine and training tools / editors, Brenda D. Carmichael and Alan B. Mitchell.
p. cm. -- (Sports and athletics preparation, performance, and psychology)
Includes bibliographical references and index.
ISBN 978-1-61122-827-4 (softcover : alk. paper)
1. Sports medicine. 2. Competency-Based Education--methods. 3. Sports injuries. I. Carmichael, Brenda D. II. Mitchell, Alan B.
RC1210.S684 2011
617.1'027--dc22
2010044754

Published by Nova Science Publishers, Inc. † New York

CONTENTS

Preface		vii
Chapter I	Wrestling with Herpes: A Case Study *John J. Miller and John T. Wendt*	1
Chapter II	Why College Athletes Play through Pain during Competition *Jennifer J. Waldron and Nathan White*	11
Chapter III	Steroids in Interscholastic Athletics: Does Reasonable Suspicion Exist? *John J. Miller, John T. Wendt and Sean Kern*	21
Chapter IV	The Importance of Parent Physical Activity Levels and Their Expectations for Their Children's Health: A Path Analysis *Marc Lochbaum, Tara Stevens, Yen To and Sarah Stevenson*	39
Chapter V	Bioenergetical Assessment and Training Control as Useful Tools to Improve Performance in Cyclic Sports *Ricardo Fernandes, Eduardo Oliveira and Paulo Colaço*	61
Chapter VI	Biomechanics of Martial Arts and Combative Sports *Osmar Pinto Neto*	89
Index		109

PREFACE

Sports medicine is an area of health and special services that apply medical and scientific knowledge to prevent, recognize, manage, and rehabilitate injuries related to sport, exercise, or recreational activity. This book examines research in the study of sports medicine, as well as training tools used to increase endurance and improve performance in athletics. Topics discussed include wrestling with herpes; steroids in interscholastic athletics; the importance of parent physical activity levels in children's health; biomechanics of martial arts; bioenergetical assessment and training control in cyclic sports and the reasons why college athletes continue to play through pain during competition.

Chapter I - A recent outbreak of herpes gladiatorum took place in a northern Midwestern state that affected 24 high school athletes from ten different schools who were diagnosed as having herpes gladiatorum (HG). In an unprecedented move the state high school league imposed a statewide shutdown of the sport for eight days in the middle of the season. A previous study indicated that not only are medical personnel not fully trained to diagnose HG but national guidelines are too lax in checking for possible symptoms for it. Because this was not the first time that such an outbreak hasd occurred in wrestling in the state, it should have been a foreseeable issue. The concepts of foreseeability, likelihood and impact will be addressed and applied to the implementation of an effective risk management plan. Through the implementation of a risk management plan such episodes as cited in the case study may be prevented from happening.

Chapter II - Within the environment of sport, athletes must often overlook and ignore pain and injury to be successful. In light of this, the current study, using an open-ended question, explored reasons why collegiate athletes made the decision to play through pain during competition. Male ($n = 67$) and female ($n = 60$) collegiate athletes from a variety of sports completed a demographic questionnaire and an open-ended question asking the reason why they played through pain during competition. Of the 127 participants, 77 (61%) reported that they had played through pain during competition. Data analysis included two researchers individually coding participants' answers. Five major labels –for the self, nature of sport, for others, pain, and self-presentation – explained why athletes' were determined to play through pain during competition. Participants' responses suggest they have internalized the norms of the sport ethic and the culture of risk.

Chapter III - Despite the notoriety that steroid use has attained, relatively little research has been conducted regarding interscholastic athletics. Miller and Wendt (2007) reported that more than twice the number of the state athletic directors perceived that steroid use was extensive throughout the United States than in their state. Additionally, the results indicated that while 40% were uncertain whether interscholastic athletes in their program had taken steroids, 25% of the athletic directors had suspected athletes is in their program had done so. Moreover, nearly 30% had suspected athletes from other athletic programs had used steroids. However, a limitation of this study was that the ascertained information came from only one state. This study expanded this number to three states. The results indicated that 33% of the respondents suspected athletes in their programs of taking steroids while 65% had suspected had suspected interscholastic athletes in other programs of taking steroids

Chapter IV - Rates of childhood obesity are reaching epidemic levels. The purpose of this investigation was to determine if parent behavior and expectations are associated with estimates of their children's leisure time activities and their adult body size. Bandura's (1986) social cognitive theory guided the investigation. Participants were 121 parents of 65 kindergarten and 56 fifth grade students from a midsized rural school district. The majority of parents were minorities with a low percentage of parents having obtained degrees beyond a high school diploma. Parents completed measures to assess their physical activity level, their preferences for their children's leisure time activity, estimates of time spent in a variety of leisure time activities, and an estimate of their children's adult body size as an adult. Parents spent very little time in physical activity though their preference was for their children to be active. Path analysis was conducted on a model that described relationships between parents' activity levels and their preferences for their children's activity, parents' activity levels and that of their children, and parents' preferences for their children's physical activity and their children's time spent in physical activity. An association was also posited between parents' preferences for their children's physical activity and their children's body size as an adult. Path analysis goodness of fit indices indicated a good fit (e.g., $SRMR = .02$, $CFI = 1.00$). All associations were in the hypothesized direction. In addition, the greater preference for children to be active was associated with a decrease in estimated body size as an adult by the parents. The percent of variance accounted for (< 10%) in the significant paths do suggest that several important variables were missing in our model. Future research longitudinal research that incorporates more extensive measures of both parents and their children are discussed.

Chapter V - Training control and evaluation of athletes are currently fundamental tools to increase the efficiency of the training process. Thus, coaches and their collaborators often implement a set of tasks that allow evaluating the level of development of the athletes' performance determinant factors as well as the result and adequacy of the training exercises and programs.

Due to their characteristics (individual, cyclic, closed and combined), several sport modalities, including running, swimming, cycling and rowing, are more prone to be evaluated. From the several determinants of the specific performance of these athletes, the bioenergetical and biomechanical factors are recognizably important and, therefore, focus of attention.

The purpose of the present chapter is to present recent data regarding bioenergetical assessment of performance in cyclic sports, giving more emphasis to running and swimming. The bioenergetical studies presented focus on the characterization of the capacity and power of the two larger body energy systems (the aerobic and the anaerobic ones) through the assessment of well-known physiological parameters like the anaerobic threshold, the maximal oxygen uptake (and the corresponding velocities) and the maximal blood lactate concentrations. Complementarily, recently proposed tests are also presented (e.g. critical velocity).

The authors hope that the presented results could be well accepted and usefull to athletes, coaches and scientists in their training control programs, helping them to increase the training efficiency and even contributing to predict performance

Chapter VI - The pioneer studies on the biomechanics of martial arts were published in the nineteen sixties and seventies. After these articles were published, several other biomechanical studies have been conducted about martial arts and other related punching sports using a variety of different measures and methods, especially in the last decade. In general, these studies were concerned with the enhancement of performance and extending the understanding of injury risk. This paper presents a comprehensive review on this subject. It is divided in two major topics: the first topic covers articles about the kinetics, kinematics and electromyography of specific hand strikes, kicks, throws and fall techniques; the second topic focus on some aspects of motor behaviors and perceptual abilities fundamental for efficient and successful performances in martial arts and combative sports (i.e. repeatability of movement, reaction time

Versions of these chapters were also published in *Journal of Contemporary Athletics* Volume 3, Numbers 1-2 and Volume 4, Number 1, edited by Dr. Dan Drane, published by Nova Science Publishers, Inc. They were submitted for appropriate modifications in an effort to encourage wider dissemination of research.

In: Sports Medicine and Training Tools
Editors: B. Carmichael and A. Mitchell

ISBN: 978-1-61122-827-4
© 2011 Nova Science Publishers, Inc.

Chapter I

WRESTLING WITH HERPES: A CASE STUDY

John J. Miller[*1] *and John T. Wendt*[2]
¹Texas Tech University
²University of St. Thomas (MN)

ABSTRACT

A recent outbreak of herpes gladiatorum took place in a northern Midwestern state that affected 24 high school athletes from ten different schools who were diagnosed as having herpes gladiatorum (HG). In an unprecedented move the state high school league imposed a statewide shutdown of the sport for eight days in the middle of the season. A previous study indicated that not only are medical personnel not fully trained to diagnose HG but national guidelines are too lax in checking for possible symptoms for it. Because this was not the first time that such an outbreak hasd occurred in wrestling in the state, it should have been a foreseeable issue. The concepts of foreseeability, likelihood and impact will be addressed and applied to the implementation of an effective risk management plan.

---

[*] Send all correspondence to: John J. Miller, Ph.D., Associate Professor, Department of Health, Exercise, and Sport Sciences, Box 41121, Texas Tech University, Lubbock, TX 79409-1121, Phone: (806) 742-3361, FAX: (806) 742-0877. Email: john.miller@ttu.edu

Through the implementation of a risk management plan such episodes as cited in the case study may be prevented from happening.

It has been acknowledged that between 60%–95% of the global population is infected by one or more viruses of the herpes family (World Health Organization, 1985). Within that family is herpes gladiatorum (HG) that was first described in the mid-1960s as a skin infection caused by the herpes simplex virus. Interscholastic athletes particularly at risk of contracting HG are often wrestlers who utilize the lock-up position, which puts the face, neck, and arms of the opposing wrestler in close contact (American College of Sport Medicine, 2003). Herpes gladiatorum causes a rash that commonly appears on the face, neck, shoulder, and arms and usually occurs when an infected wrestler passes the infection to an uninfected wrestler by skin contact (Anderson, 1999; Becker, Kodsi, Lee, Levandowski, andNahmias 1988; Whitley, Kimberlin, Roizman, 1998).

While herpes gladiatorum it is not a fatal disease, once it is contracted it becomes a permanent condition, and left untreated the infection can lead to serious consequences (Holland, Mahanti, Belongia, et al., 1992; White andGrant-Kels, 1984; Whitley, Kimberlin, Roizman, 1998). These consequences include extreme fatigue, weight loss, permanent visual impairment and conjunctivitis. Young wrestlers exhibiting symptoms such as extreme fatigue or severe weight loss could put themselves in a highly vulnerable position to incur significant injury. Moreover, some cases have been reported in which the athlete required hospitalization as a result of contracting HG (Becker, et al., 1988; Holland, Mahanti, Belongia, et al., 1992; Selling andKibrick, 1964).

Because of the extreme potential for recurrent episodes and the ease with which infection can be transmitted, the lives of students and coaches can be significantly disrupted (Maine, 2000). A disruption took place in 2007 at a northern Midwestern state as 24 high school athletes from ten different schools were diagnosed as having herpes gladiatorum. In an unprecedented move the State High School League (SHSL) declared a statewide shutdown of the sport for eight days in the middle of the season. The SHSL took the position that the shutdown was necessary for the protection of the student-athletes. The director of information for the SHSL explained,

> The safety of the states student athletes is of paramount concern; while the eight-day suspension of all wrestling competition may be considered disruptive by some, it is hoped that controlling the spread of the disease now will minimize the risk of athletes being disqualified during the upcoming section and state tournaments. The suspension period will also allow affected wrestlers to continue

their treatment as well as allow school personnel to monitor athletes that may have been exposed but who have not yet shown any symptoms (MSHSL transcript, 2007, p. 8).

Interscholastic wrestling is a major high school competition in the state as more than 7,500 interscholastic athletes from more than 250 schools annually compete (Millea, 2007).

APPLICATION OF RISK MANAGEMENT

The concept of risk management has been assigned various definitions, however, the one constant in all of these descriptions has been to prevent harm. In the context of this case study, risk management will refer to identifying foreseeable risks of contracting herpes gladiatorum through wrestling, the likelihood of occurrences, and the impact that contracting such an infectious disease may have on an individual. It is hoped that through the understanding of these ideas, effective risk management plans may be developed, implemented and enforced to avoid other interscholastic wrestlers from contracting herpes gladiatorum in the future.

Foreseeability of Risks

According to Stahl, Lichtenstein, and Mangan (2004) risks are caused by the actions of others by which a danger develops that could have been avoided. Additionally, Makropoulos (1997) promoted the idea that risks are the result of actions that are not necessary (1997). The concept of foreseeability does not address whether a harmful incident could have been averted, but whether a reasonable person could have foreseen the risks that created the incident (*Anderson v. Pine Knob Hill*, 2003).

The herpes simplex virus (HSV) infection, from which herpes gladiatorum stems, appears to be widespread among wrestlers and rugby players although no specific strain has been identified as being blamed for the outbreaks (Anderson, 2003; Dworkin, et al., 1999). According to reports from the National Federation of State High School Associations and National Collegiate Athletic Association more than 7 million athletes annually participate in interscholastic and intercollegiate athletics. As a result it is foreseeable that greater opportunities for infectious diseases to spread exist. Turbeville, Cowan, Greenfield (2006) indicated that football and wrestling were ranked first and second concerning the frequencies of sport specific outbreaks of infectious diseases. The report also revealed that contact athletics such as wrestling and rugby present tremendous environments for the transmission of communicable diseases due to the close physical contact and trauma to the skin that occurs in these sports.

Within this case study, risk was indeed a foreseeable issue as the action of an infected high school wrestler giving another competitor herpes gladiatorum. It was also unnecessary in that with proper pre-tournament inspection the infected wrestler would have been identified. Because of the prevalence of HG transmission in wrestling a pre-inspection may be considered more the norm than not, especially when the impact on the young person's life is added. Further explanation of the concepts of likelihood and impact as essential components of an effective risk management plan will be addressed in the following sections.

Likelihood

A recent report indicated that the occurrence of herpes gladiatorium escalates as the experience level of a wrestler increases, as 2.6% of all high school wrestlers, 8-13% of all in college, and 20-40% of those in Division I wrestlers have HG (StarTribune.com, 2007). While the previously described incident recently took place, it is not without a history in the state as 19 high schools sponsoring wrestling in the state's major city were caught up in a HG outbreak in 1999. The apparent genesis for the outbreak was due to a team entering a wrestling tournament, completely unaware that some of the members were infected. As a result participants on seven other teams initially contracted HG due to wrestling the infected individuals during the tournament. Additionally, it was determined that as those who were unknowingly infected as well those who became infected at the tournament continued to practice and compete afterwards. As a result the number of others who became infected increased dramatically as 61 wrestlers and three coaches were recognized as having contracted HG over a 42-day period (Anderson, 2003).

Other cases of HG outbreaks have been cited in the same state in 2000 and 2001 at summer wrestling camps (Anderson, 2003). Of the 300 wrestlers, ranging in age between 13-18 who participated in the 2000 camp, 33 or 9% of the entire camp contracted the HG infection by its completion. The origination of this outbreak stemmed from a wrestler who had a history of herpes labialis but chose not to receive suppressive therapy. In 2001, an HG outbreak took place at the same camp, however, this time 330 wrestlers between the ages of 13-18 had signed up. The wrestlers were divided into five groups of 66. Within five days of the start of the camp, three of the groups had an HG outbreak that eventually spread to members of the other groups. Eventually, 57 or 17% of the participants had contracted the HG infection by the end of camp.

The HG outbreaks that occurred in 2000 and 2001, while unfortunate, represent the foreseeability of the occurrence of herpes gladiatorum for interscholastically aged participants. As such it is the responsibility of an institution, coach or sponsoring organization to initiate procedures to protect the participants against becoming infected with HG.

Impact

The timing was critical in this case as the ban on competition extended to one week prior to sectional championships that served as the qualifying rounds to the state tournament. In other words, wrestlers were not allowed to participate in essential contact practice or competition until the week immediately preceding the qualifying rounds and championships. By preventing them from honing their skills, some young athletes may have been deprived of participating in the state tournament. For example, a coach from a team that has finished very well in recent state wrestling championships did not perceive the situation to be fair, predominately because his team did not have a recorded case of herpes (Millea, 2007). The coach continued to express concern regarding that the lack of preparation could prevent his team from doing as well as he had planned, increase the potential for injuries due to the lack of conditioning, and how this situation may affect individual's chances of obtaining an intercollegiate wrestling scholarship. Thus, the impact of HG may significantly affect the lives of young interscholastic wrestlers in potentially losing a scholarship or experiencing the thrill of participating or winning a state championship.

Another type of impact that may develop in the near future concerns potential litigation. At least one court has recognized a new tort of negligent transmission of herpes gladiatorum – that a wrestler owed another wrestler a duty based on the defendant's knowledge of his herpes blister and the degree of the skin-to-skin contact inherent in wrestling. In *Silver v. Levittown* (1999) though the court was "…loathe to create new causes of action in tort, the law must nevertheless adapt to the society in which it exists." This case was settled out of court with the defendant receiving $190,000. While not precedent setting, the Silver case may provide an insight into the potential future litigation that may occur if schools sponsoring wrestling and wrestling coaches continue to overlook infectious diseases such as herpes gladiatorum.

Implementing Procedures

The primary objective of risk management is to allow individuals and organizations to distinguish the risks into discrete categories and to identify possible alternatives to alleviate the impact of the risk. However, some of these risks may be inherent to the sport of wrestling. Risk of injury is inherent at all levels of participation in sport. Inherent risk relates to the conduct of the game and the activities that the athletes are required to do. For example, football players are expected to collide into each other to tackle and block, thus creating a potential for injury. However, to take away blocking and tackling would take away the essence of the sport. Thus, injuries due to blocking and tackling cannot be taken out of the sport of football even though they may create situations of injury.

In wrestling there are many risks that need to be attended to, such as concussions, strains, and sprains due to collisions. These risks are considered inherent to the sport of interscholastic wrestling and it is understood that they may occur through a season. However, the risk of contracting an infectious disease such as herpes gladiatorum is not one that may be considered as inherent since it is not a required activity within the sport. Yet, as explained earlier it can be a significant risk to an athlete, especially a wrestler.

During the traditional wrestling season teams often compete in dual or quadrangular meets during the week as well as weekend tournaments. As a result checks for skin lesions or abrasions that may indicate the presence of HG are sometimes not conducted prior to performed competition. In fact the National Federation for High School Sports (NFHS) guidelines do not require skin checks prior to each contest, although wrestlers found to have obvious lesions are suspended from participation supports this (NFHS, 2000).

Additionally, it is enough for a wrestler's personal physician to provide a statement that the lesion is not transmissible to allow the wrestler to compete (Anderson, 2003). However, Anderson (2003) indicated that certain factors have been shown to increase the likelihood of HG outbreaks. The primary factor cited was the dependence on the physicians of individual wrestlers to diagnose the presence of HG. Yet, many of these physicians do not understand how HG develops and spreads to others (Anderson, 2003).

The NATA has recommended that wrestling participants should shower prior and after workouts, wash workout clothes everyday, dry their skin well, avoid wearing street shoes on wrestling mats or wrestling shoes outside and conduct total body skin inspections each day. The NCAA standards also differ from the NFHS in that skin checks are recommended at all wrestling contest. Moreover, a compendium of symptoms is at hand at each contest as a criterion for withdrawal if an individual is suspected of being infected (NCAA, 2003).

Finally, NCAA guidelines recommend that only certified athletic trainers or physicians experienced in recognizing the symptoms conduct skin checks.

Conclusion

As stated earlier, the likelihood of an interscholastic wrestler contracting herpes gladiatorum is relatively high when compared to other high school sports. This is obvious within this case study as three outbreaks of HG have been cited occurring in one specific state. As a result it becomes a foreseeable risk that wrestlers, coaches, and organizations should attempt to better manage, especially since current high school guidelines seem somewhat ineffective in controlling potential HG outbreaks.

To better address such outbreaks the recommendations established by the NATA and the NCAA are excellent sources from which to develop an effective risk management plan. Secondly, increased education regarding HG and diagnosis of it of sport medicine personnel affiliated with wrestling programs is strongly encouraged. Finally, the authors encourage those involved in interscholastic wrestling to enforce a risk management plan once it has been developed. To do so may prevent a young athlete from unnecessarily contracting a disease that may affect him for the rest of his life.

References

American College of Sports Medicine. (2003). *Organization plan to reduce herpes gladiatorum outbreaks through earlier diagnosis and treatment.* Retrieved February 15, 2007, 2007, from http://www.acsm.org/AM/Template.cfm?Section=Search&template=/CM/HTMLDisplay.cfm&ContentID=4254.

Anderson, B. J. (2003). The epidemiology and clinical analysis of several outbreaks of herpes gladiatorum. *Medicine andScience in Sports andExercise, 35,* 1809-1814.

Anderson, B. J. (1999). The effectiveness of valacyclovir in preventing reactivation of herpes gladiatorum in wrestlers. *Clinical Journal of Sport Medicine, 9*, 86 - 90.

Anderson v. Pine Knob Ski Resort, Inc., 469 Mich 20, 664 N.W.2d 756 (2003).

Becker, T. M., Kodsi, P., Lee, F., Levandowski, R., andNahmias, A. J. (1988). Grappling with herpes: Herpes gladiatorum. *American Journal of Sports Medicine, 16*, 665 - 669.

Dworkin M.S., Shoemaker P.C., Spitters C., Cent, A., Hobson, A., Vieira, J., Corey, l., Frumkin, L. (1999). Endemic spread of herpes simplex virus type 1 among adolescent wrestlers and their coaches. *Pediatric Infectious Disease Journal, 18*(12), 1108-1109.

Maine Epi-Gram: Infectious Epidemiology Program. (2000). *Herpes skin infections among wrestlers: A clinician alert.* Retrieved February 15, 2007 from http://www.maine.gov/dhhs/bohepi/Jan%2000.htm#HERPES%20SKIN%20INFECTIONS%20AMONG%20WRESTLERS:%20A%20CLINICIAN%20ALERT.

Makropoulos, M. (1997). Modernitat und Kontingenz. Munich: Wilhelm Fink Verlag.

Millea, J. (2007). *7,500 state wrestlers have season put on hold.* Retrieved February 15, 2007, from http://www.startribune.com/526/story/969346.html

National Collegiate Athletic Association. (2005). *NCAA sports medicine handbook, 2005 - 2006.* Retrieved February, 15, 2007, from http://www.ncaa.org/library/sports_sciences/sports_med_handbook/2005-06/2005-06_sports_medicine_handbook.pdf

National Collegiate Athletic Association Wrestling Championships Handbook. (2003). Appendix D, WA-11-14. Indianapolis, IN.

National Federation of State High School Associations Wrestling Handbook. (2000). Rule 4-2-2, 3. Indianapolis, IN.

Simmons, A. (2002). Clinical manifestations and treatment considerations of herpes simplex virus infection. *Journal of Infectious Diseases, 186*, S71-S77.

Selling B, and Kibrick, S. (1964). An outbreak of herpes simplex among wrestlers. *New England Journal of Medicine, 270*, 979-982.

Silver v. Levittown Union Free School Dist., 692 N.Y.S.2d 886 (Sup. Ct. Nassau County 1999).

Stahl, B. C., Lichtenstein, Y., andMangan, A. (2004). The limits of risk management–a social construction approach. *Communications of the International Information Management Association, 3*(3), 15-22.

MSHSL transcript press conference. (2007). Retrieved February 15, 2007 from http://www.startribune.com/526/story/973148.html

Turbeville, S., Cowan, L., andGreenfield, R. (2006). Infectious disease outbreaks in competitive sports. *American Journal of Sports Medicine, X*(X), 1-6.

Whitley, R.J., Kimberlin, D.W., Roizman, B. (1998). Herpes simplex viruses. Clinical *Infectious Diseases, 26*, 541–53.

White, W.B., Grant-Kels, J.M. (1984). Transmission of herpes simplex virus type 1 infection in rugby players. *Journal of the American Medical Association, 252*, 533-535.

World Health Organization. (1985). Prevention and control of herpesvirus diseases (part 1). Clinical and laboratory diagnosis and chemotherapy. A WHO meeting. *Bull World Health Organization, 63*, 185 201.

In: Sports Medicine and Training Tools ISBN: 978-1-61122-827-4
Editors: B. Carmichael and A. Mitchell © 2011 Nova Science Publishers, Inc.

Chapter II

WHY COLLEGE ATHLETES PLAY THROUGH PAIN DURING COMPETITION

Jennifer J. Waldron and Nathan White
University of Northern Iowa, USA

ABSTRACT

Within the environment of sport, athletes must often overlook and ignore pain and injury to be successful. In light of this, the current study, using an open-ended question, explored reasons why collegiate athletes made the decision to play through pain during competition. Male ($n = 67$) and female ($n = 60$) collegiate athletes from a variety of sports completed a demographic questionnaire and an open-ended question asking the reason why they played through pain during competition. Of the 127 participants, 77 (61%) reported that they had played through pain during competition. Data analysis included two researchers individually coding participants' answers. Five major labels –for the self, nature of sport, for others, pain, and self-presentation – explained why athletes' were determined to play through pain during competition. Participants' responses suggest they have internalized the norms of the sport ethic and the culture of risk.

At some point in their career, most athletes will experience some pain due to injury. In order to examine the rate of injuries during practice and competition, the

National Collegiate Athletic Association (NCAA) started the Injury Surveillance System (ISS; NCAA, n. d.). Their data reveals that football players had the highest rate of injury, and collegiate injury rates were higher in competition than practice. Perception of and being able to manage pain is an important component of coping with an injury. Furthermore, many athletes are compelled to push through their pain and continue to practice or play in a competition with their pain and injury.

Both Nixon's (1992) notion of sport as a culture of risk and Coakley's (2004) concept of the sport ethic emphasize the norms and values athletes must adhere to in order to be successful. Historically, sport has been a risky venture for men as they have been encouraged to adopt a win-at-all-costs attitude. However, Waldron and Krane (2005) argue that as women gain more acceptance in the sporting environment, they too may adopt the norms and values of the sport ethic and engage in unhealthy behaviors. One of these potentially unhealthy behaviors is playing with an injury or with pain. For example, Buddy Lazier won the Indianapolis 500 in 1996 with a broken back (Coakley, 2004). This attitude was also exemplified when 29% of student athletes in a research study reported using painkilling drugs to cope with pain during competition was an acceptable action (Tricker, 2000). Within the environment of sport, athletes must often overlook and ignore pain and injury to be successful.

Previous theorists have suggested that collegiate men and women may respond to athletic injuries differently (Wiese-Bjornstal and Shaffer, 1999). For example, female athletes, compared to male athletes, were more concerned about how the coach treated them after the injury and how the injury would influence their future health (Granito, 2002). Thus, it is possible that female athletes have different reasons for playing through pain than their male counterparts. Research with a youth corecreational basketball league determined that boys, as compared to girls, were held to a more limiting criterion of how to correctly respond to pain (Singer, 2004). Therefore, the purpose of the current study was to explore, using an open-ended question, reasons why collegiate athletes made the decision to play through pain during competition. Additionally, we examined gender differences in the reasons why athletes play through pain. It was hypothesized that a relationship between gender and reason for playing through pain exists.

METHOD

Participants and Procedures

After Institutional Review Board approval, coaches of collegiate teams were contacted to set up times for administration of the questionnaires to athletes.

Male ($n = 67$) and female ($n = 60$) collegiate athletes from a variety of sports (e.g., softball, basketball, swimming, and wrestling) completed a demographic questionnaire as well as an open-ended question asking the top three reasons they decided to play through pain during competition. Of the 127 participants, 77 (61%) reported that they had played through pain during competition and 28 (36%) of the 77 had sustained further injury.

Thus, data analysis was based on the 77 participants who had competed with pain during competition. Seventy-seven participants responded with a top reason, 69 participants responded with a second reason, and 61 participants responded with a third reason for playing through pain during competition.

Data Analysis

In order to examine reasons athletes played through pain, data analysis included two researchers individually coding participants' responses. A reliability coefficient was calculated using a percentage (Granito, 2002). That is, the number of coded agreements between the two researchers for the first, second, and third response was divided by the total number of respective responses. The reliability coefficient ranged from 89% to 95%. Five major labels and nine minor labels emerged from the data and explained why athletes' were determined to play through pain during competition.

To facilitate the examination of gender differences, each athlete's response was entered into the Statistical Package for the Social Sciences (SPSS). That is, the nine minor labels (e.g., desire, win, team) for the first, second, and third reason were coded for each participant. A chi-square test for independence was then conducted to determine if there was a relationship between gender and reason for playing through pain.

RESULTS

Results showed that athletes competed with pain for a variety of reasons. Specifically, five major labels and nine minor labels emerged for why athletes play through pain during competition (see Table 1). Of the 77 participants who competed with pain during competition, 24 (31.1%) reported the top reason was for themselves. Some of the athletes proposed that they competed with pain due to their own desire; for example, athletes stated they "wanted and needed to," "would regret not trying," and "had never quit anything in my life." The other athletes reported their need to display continual effort and improvement in sport. Among these responses, athletes detailed wanting the "opportunity to play," "doing well," and "reach my goals."

Within the first reason, 21 (27.2%) of the athletes reported they decided to play through pain because of the nature of the sport. For example, intracollegiate competition ("proving I am worth what I get paid to do," and "fight for spot"), intercollegiate competition ("it was nationals" and "end of season"), and winning reflected the nature of sport. Nineteen (24.6%) of the played with pain because other people. Overwhelmingly, athletes were compelled to play through pain because of their teammates, while a couple of athletes played because of their parents and coaches. Common responses included, "didn't want to let team down," "wanted to help team," and "team needed me." Finally, 13 (16.8%) of the athletes reported playing with pain during competition because of the nature of their pain. For example, athletes expressed that the "pain was bearable," that they had "done it before," or that they were "physically able to."

The second and third reasons for playing through pain during competition reported by athletes closely reflected the first reason specified above with one exception. Both the second and third reasons included a category labeled presentation to the team, where athletes wanted to portray a certain image to their teammates, coaches, or fans. Namely, athletes "didn't want teammates to look down on me," "show was tough," or "didn't want to be seen as weak."

A second purpose of the current study was to examine if gender differences existed among the reported responses. To answer this question, a chi-square analysis was conducted for the nine minor labels emerging from the first, second, and third reason. No significant gender differences were revealed within the first, $\chi^2(8, n = 77) = 7.19, p = .52$, or the second reason, $\chi^2(9, n = 69) = 12.38, p = .19$.

Table 1. Major and Minor Labels for First, Second, and Third Reason for Playing with Pain during Competition

Major and Minor Labels	First Reason			Second Reason			Third Reason		
	Men	Women	Total	Men	Women	Total	Men	Women	Total
For Self	12	12	24	7	15	23	12	11	23
Desire	7	8	15	7	12	19	11	6	17
Effort and Improvement	5	4	9	1	3	4	1	5	6
Nature of Sport	13	8	21	3	3	6	7	2	9
Intracollegiate Competition	4	5	9	0	1	1	0	2	2
Win	4	2	6	1	1	2	3	0	3
Intercollegiate Competition	5	1	6	2	1	3	4	0	4
For Others	9	10	19	7	11	18	3	7	10
Team	8	9	17	6	9	15	3	6	9
Parents and Coaches	1	1	2	2	1	3	0	1	1
Pain	7	6	13	13	3	16	4	7	11
Bearing Pain	6	2	8	12	2	14	4	5	9
Lack of Pain	1	4	5	1	1	2	0	1	1
Presentation to the Team	0	0	0	2	4	6	6	3	9

However, a significant gender difference was found in the third reason reported for playing through pain during competition, χ^2 (9, n = 61) = 18.07, p = .034. Upon closer examination, more men than expected provided reasons within the minor labels of intercollegiate competition (end of the season, for my record, etc.), wanting to win, and team presentation, while women were overrepresented in the minor label of competing for the team.

DISCUSSION

Previous research has found that a majority of athletes believe that an athlete has to be willing to accept risks (Nixon, 1993). One of these risks is playing with pain and injury during competition. In the current study, 61% of the participants admitted to and justified why they decided to compete with pain. This suggests that the athletes had been socialized to value the culture of risk or the sport ethic. In the current study, the most frequent reported motivation was for reasons concerning the self, including desire and effort and improvement. This category indicates that athletes have internalized the importance of being competitive, having pride, and loving their sport uncritically to such an extent that they are willing to play through pain.

Many athletes also responded that they were motivated to compete with pain because of the nature of sport. That is, the structural support for playing with pain, such as recognition and financial rewards (Nixon, 2004), encourage some athletes to play through pain. Teammates, and to a lesser degree coaches and parents, also place covert pressure on athletes. Many athletes believe that if they refused to play with an injury they would be letting their teammates down. Similarly, Charlesworth and Young (2004) reported that the most frequent motivator reported by English, female, university athletes for playing with an injury was not wanting to let down their teammates.

A number of athletes also commented that they often could withstand the pain while they were playing or had play with pain in the past. Essentially, athletes have learned the culture of risk and injury. Within this culture, they ignore pain and continue to play with the pain even though this decision may result in further injury. Although the lowest number of responses emerged from the team presentation category, it is an intriguing category. Some athletes were concerned that they would present the wrong image to their teammates if they did not play in pain. In other words, athletes wanted to show their toughness and prove they were truly deserving of the athlete label.

The second purpose of the research was to examine gender differences in the responses that male and female athletes give for playing through pain. Counter to the hypothesis, the chi-square analysis revealed no differences between the first and second responses given by men and women. The observed number of responses for the first and second reasons from men and women matched the expected number for each minor label. However, the chi-square analysis uncovered a significant gender difference in the third reason given for playing through pain. Specifically, men were overrepresented in the minor labels of intercollegiate competition (end of the season, for my record, etc.), wanting to win, and team presentation, while women were overrepresented in the minor label of competing for the team.

Both men and women appear to possess similar motives for playing through pain during competition. This would provide evidence that women are adopting the norms and values of the sport ethic (Waldron and Krane, 2005). Gender differences did not emerge until the third reason given by the athletes. Gender differences revealed in the minor labels of the third reason reflects, to some degree, gender norms and stereotypes in our society. Gender stereotypes often suggest that women, as compared to men, value interpersonal relationships or living connected to others (DeBoer, 2004). Within the third reason, more women than expected replied they played through pain because of their teammates, which reflects the stereotype of women. On the other hand gender stereotypes often imply that men, as compared to women, do not want to be helpless and are concerned with proving themselves (DeBoer, 2004). It follows, then, that men were overrepresented in the minor labels of intercollegiate competition, wanting to win, and team presentation.

There are limitations to the current study. Neither pain perceptions nor examination of different pain experiences of the athletes were measured. First, individual athletes may perceive pain differently. For example, catastrophizing via rumination, intensification, and helplessness is associated with increased pain (Sullivan, Tripp, Rodgers, and Stanish, 2000). If pain perception was accounted for, it is possible that the findings would change. Second, pain in sport can stem from the training aspects or actual injury. Participants in the current study were specifically asked about pain caused from injury; however, Safai (2003) argues that in the sport culture athletes are not taught to distinguish one pain from the other. Therefore, it is possible that some athletes responded in terms of pain from training aspects rather than actual injury. Future research could examine the relationship between pain perception or different types of pain and athletes' motivations for playing with pain

The current study contributes to the larger literature examining pain, injury, and gender. From athletes' responses to an open-ended question, five major and nine minor labels emerged for why they played through pain. Additionally, very few gender differences emerged regarding motives for playing through pain. In particular, the findings suggest that collegiate athletes were socialized into the culture of sport and were willing to accept risks associated with being an athlete. When embedded in the culture of sport, it may be difficult for an athlete to assess when acceptance of risk and playing through pain is resulting in damage to one's body, health, and well being. As practitioners working with athletes, it is crucial that we understand this culture of risk and the sport ethic to help athletes avoid long term damage to their health.

REFERENCES

Charlesworth, H., and Young, K. (2004). Why English female university athletes play with pain: Motivations and rationalisations. In K. Young (Ed.), *Sporting bodies, damaged selves*. (pp.163-180). Boston: Elsevier.

Coakley, J. (2004). *Sports in society: Issues and controversies* (8th ed.). Boston: McGraw-Hill.

DeBoer, K. J. (2004). *Gender and competition: How men and women approach work and play differently*. Monterey, NJ: Coaches Choice.

Granito, V. J. (2002). Psychological response to athletic injury: Gender differences. *Journal of Sport Behavior, 25,* 243-260.

National Collegiate Athletic Association Retrieved April 17, 2007, from http://www1.ncaa.org/membership/ed_outreach/health-safety/iss/index.html

Nixon, H. L. (1992). A Social Network Analysis of Influences on Athletes to Play With Pain and Injuries. *Journal of Sport and Social Issues, 16*(2), 127-135.

Nixon, H. L. (1993). Accepting the risks of pain and injury in sport: Mediated cultural influences on playing hurt. *Sociology of Sport Journal, 10,* 183-196.

Nixon, H. L., (1996). Explaining pain and injury attitudes and experiences in sport in terms of gender, race, and sports status factors. *Journal of Sport and Social Issues, 20*(1), 33-44.

Nixon, H. L. (2004). Cultural, structural, and status dimensions of pain and injury experiences in sport. In K. Young (Ed.), *Sporting bodies, damaged selves*. (pp. 81-97). Boston: Elsevier.

Safai, P. (2003). Healing the body in the "culture of risk": Examining the negotiation of treatment between sport medicine clinicians and injured athletes in intercollegiate sport. *Sociology of Sport Journal, 20,* 127-164.

Singer, R. L. (2004). Pain and injury in a youth recreational basketball league. In K. Young (Ed.), *Sporting bodies, damaged selves.* (pp. 223-235). Boston: Elsevier.

Sullivan, M. J. L., Tripp, D. A., Rodgers, W. M., and Stanish, W. (2000). Catastrophizing and pain perception in sport participants. *Journal of Applied Sport Psychology, 12,* 151-167.

Tricker, R. (2000). Painkilling drugs in collegiate athletics: Knowledge, attitudes, and use of student athletes. *Journal of Drug Education, 30,* 313-324.

Waldron, J. J., and Krane, V. (2005). Whatever it takes: Health compromising behaviors in female athletes. *Quest, 57,* 315-329.

Wiese-Bjornstal, D., and Shaffer, S. (1999). Psychosocial dimensions of sport injury. In R. Ray and D. Wiese-Bjornstal (Eds.), *Counseling in sport medicine.* (pp. 23-40). Champaign, IL: Human Kinetics.

In: Sports Medicine and Training Tools
Editors: B. Carmichael and A. Mitchell

ISBN: 978-1-61122-827-4
© 2011 Nova Science Publishers, Inc.

Chapter III

STEROIDS IN INTERSCHOLASTIC ATHLETICS: DOES REASONABLE SUSPICION EXIST?

John J. Miller[*1], *John T. Wendt*[2] *and Sean Kern*[3]

[1]Texas Tech University, USA
[2]University of St. Thomas (MN), USA
[3]Texas Tech University, USA

ABSTRACT

Despite the notoriety that steroid use has attained, relatively little research has been conducted regarding interscholastic athletics. Miller and Wendt (2007) reported that more than twice the number of the state athletic directors perceived that steroid use was extensive throughout the United States than in their state. Additionally, the results indicated that while 40% were uncertain whether interscholastic athletes in their program had taken steroids, 25% of the athletic directors had suspected athletes is in their program had done so. Moreover, nearly 30% had suspected athletes from other athletic programs had used steroids. However, a limitation of this study

---

[*] Send all correspondence to: John J. Miller, Ph.D., Associate Professor, Department of Health, Exercise, and Sport Sciences, Box 41121, Texas Tech University, Lubbock, TX 79409-1121, Phone: (806) 742-3361, FAX: (806) 742-0877; Email: john.miller@ttu.edu

was that the ascertained information came from only one state. This study expanded this number to three states. The results indicated that 33% of the respondents suspected athletes in their programs of taking steroids while 65% had suspected had suspected interscholastic athletes in other programs of taking steroids

Evidence about performance-enhancing drugs, specifically anabolic steroids abounds in many recent news reports. While most of the media reports have been on professional sports, another area of focus is developing in interscholastic athletics (Latiner, 2006; Miller and Wendt, 2007). This attention is not unwarranted as interscholastic athletes have been caught using steroids in Texas and Arizona, among other states (Dickerson, 2005; Moore, 2005). Additionally, the commissioner of the Florida High School Athletic Association stated that, "You begin to worry about how widespread the problem is at the professional level. You know that there has to be a trickle-down effect when it comes to that, and that would be to the colleges and high schools" (Kallestad, 2005).

For many high school athletes the drive to win, sometimes at all costs, is all encompassing. Aside from bragging rights and personal satisfaction, a young athlete may be driven to obtaining a Division I scholarship or professional contract. To achieve such goals, athletes may incorporate supplements and performance-enhancing drugs into their training. According to an Arizona high school athlete, "The people who just have natural talent and work really hard almost can't compete. You're either really gifted or taking steroids to get really mean and strong" (Dickerson, 2005).

Devoid of any consequences, a potential message being sent is that performance enhancing drugs such as steroids are essential to achieve success. This perception was very evident as a young athlete confessed to his father just prior to committing suicide that was linked to steroid use:

> I'm on steroids, what do you think? Who do you think I am? I'm a baseball player, baseball players take steroids. How do you think Bonds hits all his home runs? How do you think all these guys do all this stuff? You think they do it from just working out normal? (Fainaru-Wada, 2004, p. 1A).

ESTIMATED NUMBER OF STEROID USERS IN HIGH SCHOOL

It has been estimated that 1 to 3 million athletes in the United States had taken steroids (Silver, 2001). Another study by Blue Cross/Blue Shield (2003) indicated more than 1 million adolescents between the ages of 12-17 had taken performance-enhancing supplements and drugs. A more significant result of the study revealed that all youths surveyed knew someone using performance-enhancing substances such as steroids. A 2002 study by Texas AandM University estimated that up to 42,000 Texas high school aged students were abusing steroids (Livingstone, 2005). An investigation by the American College of Sports Medicine (ACSM) (2004) stated that more than one out of every ten students in the United States would have used steroids by 2010. The Center for Disease Control and Prevention (CDC) (2004) has indicated that illegal steroid use between ninth through twelfth grade students has more than doubled in the last decade from 2.7% in 1991 to 6.1% in 2003. Another study by the CDC illustrated an alarming steroid use of adolescents in which 11.2% of high school males in Louisiana and 5.7% of high school girls in Tennessee had taken steroids (Office of the National Drug Control Policy, 2005).

While these reports point toward the potential likelihood of the use of steroids by high school students, they may identify the proverbial "tip of the iceberg" for steroid use in interscholastic sports. Moreover, it is alarming that significantly few high school students perceive steroids as being harmful (Johnston, O'Malley, Bachman, and Schulenberg, 2003). "Everyone knows it, but they hide it. It's a win-win situation for everybody, so no one's going to admit anything" (Dickerson, 2005).

STATE STEROID TESTING LEGISLATION

In response to testing interscholastic athletes for steroids a Michigan legislator stated, "Is it a problem right now? I think we're naive to think that it's not with the competitive nature of sports, especially among the kids who want to go on to the next level" (States consider high school steroid testing, 2005). It has been reported that 13% of high schools test for drugs nationally, but less than one-third of those schools test for steroids (National Federation of State High School Associations, 2003). Despite this traditional practice, some states (New Jersey,

Florida and Texas) and counties (Polk County, Florida) have recently enacted legislation requiring interscholastic athletes to submit to steroid testing (Moore, 2005).

New Jersey was the first state to implement drug testing for steroids on the high school level at an estimated cost of $100,000. On December 20, 2005 then acting Governor Richard Codey, by Executive Order, directed the New Jersey Department of Education to work with the New Jersey Interscholastic Athletic Association (NJSIAA),

> "... to develop and implement a program of random testing for steroids of teams and individuals qualifying for championship games" to commence with the 2006-2007 school year" (State of New Jersey, 2005). Under the NJSIAA plan, the high school league randomly tested approximately 500 student athletes that qualified for state championship tournaments or competition, primarily in football, wrestling, baseball, track and field, swimming and diving, and lacrosse (NJSIAA Steroid FAQ, 2007).

It is interesting that NJSIAA mandated that no student may participate in NJSIAA competition unless the student and their parent/guardian signed a random testing consent form. The consent form stipulated that if the student or the student's team qualified for a state tournament, the participant may be subject to testing for banned substances (NJSIAA Policy, 2007). If a student-athlete tests positive for steroid use the penalty for such an offense is a one year suspension.

In 2007 the Florida State Legislature allocated $100,000 for the testing and ordered the Florida High School Athletic Association (FHSAA) to facilitate a one year anabolic steroid testing program (2007-08) for students in grades 9 through 12 who participate in boy's football, girls' flag football, girls' softball, boys' baseball, or boys' and girls' weightlifting (Florida Statutes, 2007). State Representative Marcelo Llorente, the bill's sponsor, said that those sports were chosen because they are sports where muscle mass most enhances performance (Kallestad, 2007).

Under the Florida plan each student-athlete who participated in the identified sport, was required to sign a consent form (FHSAA Consent Form, 2007). It was estimated that 59,000 Florida high school students who participated in one of the three sports would be affected and be required to submit to random drug tests under the bill (Bender, 2007). If a student-athlete tested positive for steroids, a 90 day suspension penalty would be assessed.

Texas has perhaps the most ambitious plan as the state legislature allocated an estimated at $3 million to implement high school steroid testing policies and procedures. As a result, the Texas University Interscholastic League (UIL), which governs interscholastic athletics, plans to test a minimum 3% of the approximately of the 740,000 student athletes students who participate in UIL athletic activities annually. To put this number into perspective, the three percent of the 740,000 represents 22,000 high school students which is more than those tested in the NCAA and Olympics from 2004 (International Herald Tribune, 2007).

Under the Texas program each student and their parent/guardian agrees that as a prerequisite to participation in UIL athletic activities, they will, if selected, submit to steroid testing. As opposed to the three month suspension that a Florida athlete who tests positive would have to serve, the consequences in Texas are more severe. For example, the punishment for the first time an athlete tests positive for steroids is a 30 day suspension. If that same student-athlete tests positive a second time a one year ban is assessed. Finally, a third time offender will be banned from any type of competition for the remainder of his/her career.

The Texas testing protocol was scheduled to begin before the high school football season ended in the fall of 2007. However, it is still in the review process. UIL spokeswoman Kim Rogers said,

> "We don't know when it will begin and when it will end." Texas State Representative Dan Flynn, House sponsor of Senate Bill 8, which created the $3 million a year steroid-testing program said, "Nothing has happened. Football season is over, and we did not test one kid" (Sharrer, 2007).

REASONABLE SUSPICION

With all of the concern surrounding who might be taking steroids, the concept of reasonable suspicion may occur. Reasonable suspicion may be regarded as the degree of knowledge that would cause a reasonable person, under similar circumstances, to believe a student-athlete is involved in using or abusing a banned substance. In such cases an athletic director, athletic trainer, or coach may request a drug test. As a result, school officials need only have reasonable suspicion that a particular test will verify that a student-athlete has violated or is violating the law (Shulter, 1996; Yamaguchi, O'Malley, and Johnston, 2004; Zirkel, 2000).

Although reasonable suspicion may be present, to be permissible, the scope of the search must be such that the measures used are reasonably related to the purpose of the search, and not excessively intrusive in light of the age and gender of the student and the nature of the suspected infraction. The *New Jersey v. T.L.O* (1985) court stated,

> A school official may properly conduct a search of a student's person if the official has a reasonable suspicion that a crime has been or is in the process of being committed or reasonable cause to believe that the search is necessary to maintain school discipline or enforce school policies. (*New Jersey v. T.L.O.*, p. 329, 1985).

In *Schaill v. Tippecanoe County School Corporation* (1988) the court held that the school's interest in protecting health, safety, and integrity of sport and school outweighed an athlete's diminished expectations of privacy. In *Schaill*, the school board chose to employ a random drug-testing program for all extracurricular participants including interscholastic athletes and cheerleaders. The court reported the drug testing policy to be reasonable because it was commonly conducted in intercollegiate athletics and Olympic sports. Moreover, the students had previously consented to the testing procedure.

Drug testing of a student by a public school official is a search that must adhere to the stipulations of the Fourth Amendment that prohibits all unreasonable searches and seizures by state officers. Reasonableness is determined by balancing the governmental interest behind the search against the privacy intrusion of the search. Generally, courts have ruled that drug testing for athletic teams is allowed due to a diminished expectation of privacy of a student-athlete. For example, it is not uncommon for student-athletes to disrobe in front of others or use communal showers after a practice or game. Because these are normal practices the courts have reported that those who choose to participate in interscholastic sports have a diminished expectation of privacy (Knapp, 1990).

The court in *Vernonia v. Acton* (1995) indicated that urine collection and testing compromised a search. To determine the constitutionality of searches, three steps are required. The first aspect to be considered is whether a search and seizure was conducted by a government entity. The second step needs to identify if the officials have the power to conduct the search. The third piece addresses whether the search was reasonable depending upon the type of search.

In shaping the idea of reasonableness in searching high school students the Supreme Court stated that:

> The legality of a search of a student should depend simply on the reasonableness, under all the circumstances, of the search. Determining the reasonableness of any search involves a twofold inquiry: first, one must consider whether the action was justified at its inception, second, one must determine

whether the search as actually conducted was reasonably related in scope to the circumstances which justified the interference in the first place. Under ordinary circumstances, a search of a student by a teacher or other school official will be justified at its inception when there are reasonable grounds for suspecting that the search will turn up evidence that the student has violated or is violating either the law or the rules of the school (*New Jersey v. T.L.O.*, 1985, p. 341).

While upholding the drug testing policy in *Vernonia* (1995), the Supreme Court balanced the school's interest in conducting the drug test against the privacy interest upon which the test intrudes. In the Court's opinion, safety risks were especially great in sports:

> Finally, it must not be lost sight of that this program is directed more narrowly to drug use by school athletes, where the risk of immediate physical harm to the drug user or those with whom he is playing his sport is particularly high. Apart from psychological effects, which include impairment of judgment, slow reaction time, and a lessening of the perception of pain, the particular drugs screened by the District's Policy have been demonstrated to pose substantial physical risks to athletes (p. 661).

Finally, the *Board of Education v. Earls* (2002) permitted urinalysis drug testing for all high school extracurricular participants. By doing so, the *Earls* decision expanded the scope identified in *Vernonia* by permitting a school district to test high school students with less of a foundation.

PURPOSE OF THE STUDY

Despite the notoriety that steroid use has attained, relatively little research has been conducted regarding interscholastic athletics. Miller and Wendt (2007) reported that more than twice the number of the state athletic directors perceived that steroid use was extensive throughout the United States than in their state. Additionally, the results indicated that while 40% were uncertain whether interscholastic athletes in their program had taken steroids, 25% of the athletic directors had suspected athletes is in their program had done so. Moreover, nearly 30% had suspected athletes from other athletic programs had used steroids. However, a limitation of this study was that the ascertained information came from only one state. Thus, it is the purpose of this study to determine the level, if any, of interscholastic directors in multiple states of suspecting student-athletes of using steroids.

METHOD

Design and Procedure

The authors for this investigation developed a 1-5 Likert scale 20-item questionnaire. The Likert scale responses ranged from 1=strongly agree, 2=agree, 3=unsure, 4=disagree, and 5=strongly disagree. The questionnaire consisted of sections relating to the following areas: demographic information, suspicion of interscholastic athlete use of steroids, reasons for the suspicions.

In order to ensure the reliability of the questionnaire, a test-retest protocol was conducted with two present and three retired high school athletic directors. Several changes to the questionnaire regarding item inclusion and item wording were suggested and implemented. The re-test was accomplished two weeks later with the same group of professionals and no additional modifications were recommended. To determine the validity of the instrument, a Pearson product-moment correlation coefficient (Pearson's r) was employed. The reliability coefficient was determined to be .78, which is well within the acceptable range for the interpretation of scores for individuals (Patten, 2000).

The population for this study was 345 randomly selected interscholastic athletic directors from three states. One state is located in the southwestern part of the United States, the second is located in the mid-south, and the third is located in the upper Midwest. To maintain confidentiality, all surveys were sent en masse and all results were accumulated using a SelectSurvey ASP online survey tool. Thus, those specific individuals who completed and returned the survey could not be determined thereby ensuring anonymity and confidentiality.

After the initial email, 63 responses were received indicating that the individual was no longer at that address. To ensure that all representatives were given an opportunity to participate in this study, one of the investigators went to the each school's website to determine if that person was still employed at the school. If another individual had become the athletic director a survey was electronically sent to that individual. If no response had been received after one week following the initial contact, a follow-up email was sent. In 15 cases, the email address of the athletic director no longer appeared thus the total population of the study was 330. Of the 330 athletic directors contacted, 117 (35%) from three states responded to the online survey. Even though the investigators had hoped for a higher return, the response rate was within the parameters for effective online surveys (Paolo, Bonaminio, Gibson, Patridge, and Kallail, 2000).

RESULTS

Demographic Information

A demographic breakdown of the respondents revealed that 44 (38%) resided in the mid-South, 39 (33%) from the Southwest, and 34 (29%) from the upper Midwest. Occupationally, 71 (61%) had been an athletic director for 1-5 years. This result corresponds to the finding that 64 (55%) had been at their present position for 1-5 years. Seventy-three (62%) of the respondents reported that they were reasonably knowledgeable about interscholastic sports, including the ability to identify symptoms of steroid use. For this study, a reasonably knowledgeable person was one who understood all aspects of interscholastic sports. Thus, it appeared that the majority of respondents were well-informed regarding steroids but relatively new in interscholastic athletic administration.

Suspicion of Athletes Taking Steroids

The athletic directors were asked if they had reason to suspect interscholastic athletes in their own programs of using steroids. While 64 (55%) did not suspect their athletes of steroid use it is noteworthy that 39 (33%) had suspected such a practice. Interestingly, 76 (65%) had suspected interscholastic athletes in other programs of taking steroids and 23 (20%) did not.

To determine if any relationships existed among the states, a Pearson r correlation was employed ($p=.05$). The results indicated a significant relationship ($p=.008$) appeared between the states and athletic directors who suspected athletes in other interscholastic programs of using steroids. Although a relationship between states and suspecting their own athletes of taking steroids did not meet the established level of significance, a correlation of .074 pointed towards the significant level.

The respondents were given opportunities to provide open-ended answers for their suspicions. The primary reasons given were extraordinary gains in size (82%), perceived strength (78%), speed (73%), or a combination (68%). Also, such items as increased aggression, unexplainable facial hair and/or deepened voice were cited as reasons for suspicion. Finally, the population was asked to identify the gender of the student-athlete(s) they had suspected. More than 97% male and approximately 2% female were identified.

DISCUSSION

The use of performance enhancing drugs is not a new trend (Bahrke and Yesalis, 2002). For example, the winner of the 1904 Olympic marathon purportedly received an injection of the performance-enhancing drug, strychnine, while the race was occurring. However, the performance enhancing abilities of today's drugs are much more advanced and effective today than in the days of strychnine. Current media coverage has created a greater awareness of performance enhancement drug from the general public to the governing bodies of sport. The issue of performance enhancing drugs, especially anabolic steroids has attracted worldwide attention.

Taking steroids to enhance athletic performance is not a new topic in interscholastic sports. This history can be traced back to the early 1950s during which Russian Olympic athletes started to outperform their counterparts from the United States due to steroid use. Soon thereafter a physician associated with the U.S. Olympic team worked with chemists to create the steroid Dianabol for the Americans (McDevitt, 1994). The use of steroids spread to the point that the first documented case of a high school football athlete taking steroids to improve his performance in the late 1950's (Sturmi and Diorio, 1998).

While the use of performance enhancing drugs such as steroids have attained notoriety in professional sports, the use of such drugs in interscholastic athletics is of significant concern today since about 57% of all high school students play on formal sports teams (Grunbaum, Kann, Kinchen, Ross, Hawkins, Lowry, Harris, McManus, Chyen, and Collins, 2004). Yet, the results of a national survey revealed that less than 30% of high schools had tested for steroids (National Federation of State High School Associations, 2003).

While many question the effectiveness and legality of steroid testing, Frank Uryasz, president of the National Center for Drug Free Sport, has stated that testing ultimately will be needed to put teeth into any anti-steroid plan (Moore, 2005). Even the United States Olympic Committee has taken notice. USOC spokesman Darryl Seibel said,

> The high school athletic associations and the legislatures are absolutely doing the right thing by taking a serious look at this problem. The reported rates of steroid use at the high school level are not only alarming, they reveal the extent to which this is becoming a societal problem" (Pells, 2007).

For testing to occur, however, reasonable suspicion needs to exist. The concept of reasonable suspicion, as put forth by the U.S. Supreme Court, requires significantly more substantiation than mere curiosity, rumor or general suspicion. Items that have been recognized by courts for searching a student include observing particular and quantifiable behavior that would lead a reasonably knowledgeable professional to believe that a student is engaged or has engaged in illicit behavior. While a previous study has indicated relatively few interscholastic directors have been reported to be knowledgeable about performance-enhancing drugs (Tokish, Kocher, and Hawkins, 2004), they possess a duty to diminish exposing an athlete to foreseeable harm, including ingesting illegal substances (Heckman, 2000).

The results of this study indicate that the majority of athletic directors have suspected athletes in other programs of being "on" steroids. The reasons for their suspicion such as extraordinary gains in size, strength, speed or a combination have been recognized as potential symptoms of steroid use (Bhasin, Storer, Berman, et al., 1996; Miller, 2000; National Institute on Drug Abuse [NIDA], 2004). Also, such items as increased aggression, unexplainable facial hair and/or deepened voice appear to be valid symptoms of steroid use (Pope, Kouri, and Hudson, 2000). While it is interesting that the majority of respondents believed that "others athletes" were taking steroids, it is noteworthy that one-third of the athletic directors believed that some their "own athletes" had taken steroids.

To make doubt tangible, school officials may consider testing student-athletes for steroids under the auspices of reasonable suspicion. A primary criticism of steroid testing in interscholastic athletics is that only a few athletes will be submitted to them. For example, in New Jersey only the athletes on teams competing in the state final will be asked for a steroid test. As a result some, if not many, of the offenders may avoid detection due to prior knowledge of when a test might occur. Yet, Robert DuPont, president of the Institute for Behavior and Health and first director of the National Institute on Drug Abuse, recently described the need for drug testing in high schools,

> The schools that have, at least the ones that I know who have used random student drug testing, are all convinced that it makes a big difference in the quality of the school life. One study done by Linn Goldberg found that when he compared athletes in two schools, one that used student drug testing and one that didn't, and the school that did use the drug testing had one-quarter the drug use of the school that was not using drug testing. I don't know whether it reduced it by 75%, which is what the study found, but it surely does. And it flies in the face of reason to think it wouldn't. It would be a little bit like arguing that if you enforce the speed limit on the highway, won't slow down. That fact is that when there is a reason not to use, in this case random student drug testing, the students do less drugs (Justice Talking, 2006).

Conclusion

This study should not be construed as advocating for testing as the only method to curb steroid use in interscholastic athletics. In fact, the authors have previously proposed a three-step approach to limit the use of steroids in interscholastic athletics. The proposal included mandating administrators or others in charge of extracurricular activities to become knowledgeable about performance enhancing drugs such as steroids; educating the student-athlete about the consequences of taking steroids; and incorporating random steroid drug testing for interscholastic athletics.

There is a serious question about the efficacy to which testing is successful in decreasing the use of performance-enhancing substances, as opposed to merely generating new ways to avoid detection. For example, in cases when testing occurred for announced, in-season or unannounced, out-of-competition training the results indicated that users were not being identified (Jacobs and Samuels, 1994). However, it should be pointed out that these tests were being conducted on older professional or Olympic athletes who had the knowledge and wherewithal to avoid detection. It may be reasonable to believe that most interscholastic athletes do not adequately possess the background or information to mask taking the substance.

Presently, only New Jersey, Florida and Texas have passed state legislation requiring high school students to submit to drug testing for steroids. Steroid testing in interscholastic activities has even received attention from the White House. In October, 2007 John Walters, Director of National Drug Control Policy (ONDCP) (2007), hailed the results of New Jersey's plan as a successful example of preventing drug use among youth,

> Results from New Jersey's steroid testing program demonstrate the immense prevention power of random student testing and should provide an impetus for other communities to consider implementing programs of their own. Building on the success of this program, New Jersey and other States with steroid testing programs should consider expanding the random drug tests to include other drugs commonly abused by young people, like marijuana and prescription pain killers (White House Office of National Drug Control Policy, 2007).

One of the problems of these steroid testing policies has been that only a few athletes would be selected to take the test and only after a championship. For example, according to the New Jersey State Interscholastic Athletic Association only one high school athlete out of 500 tested positive for steroid use during the testing process. This type of suspicionless random testing, however, may permit those who had taken steroids to "slip through the cracks" by not being selected. This argument provides even greater fodder for state high school associations to increase the educational process of athletic administrators, coaches, and athletes so as to better understand the symptoms and consequences of steroid use. The results of this study revealed that athletic directors suspected that athletes, primarily from other teams, had used steroids at the interscholastic level. Although some may perceive this information as simple allegations against the competition, the fact that many of the respondents recognized several valid symptoms of steroid use is important to note. Additionally, it is significant that a majority of the respondents felt confident in recognizing the signs of steroid use. It is hoped that through this increased knowledge that athletic administrators will have an even greater basis on which to reasonably suspect steroid use in interscholastic athletics.

It has been alleged that drug-testing procedures violate a student-athlete's their right of privacy and breaches their right to participate, yet, the courts have held that participation in sports is considered a privilege and not a right (*Palmer v. Merluzzi*, 1988). The implementation of random suspicionless drug-testing of interscholastic athletes may have a significant outcome on thwarting or decreasing steroid use. If those in charge of the program suspect that interscholastic athletes of taking steroids, the need for testing along with education, is clear.

Since high school is a place where adolescent patterns develop that may lead into adulthood, it should be the first place that school officials make certain that student are aware of the consequences of taking illicit drugs such as steroids (*Vernonia v. Acton*, 1995). The Supreme Court has stated the safety of students to be a valid government interest that outweighs the students' constitutional protection from unreasonable searches and seizures (*Board of Education v. Earls*, 2002; *Vernonia v. Acton*, 1995).

It would be logical, therefore, for the Supreme Court to authorize testing in high schools for performance-enhancing drugs, as long as the privacy and safety of the students are considered. It is also true that the steroid use may immediately present a risk to the health and safety of the student-athlete, but those risks may be judged to be within acceptable limits than the risk of losing a game, championship or scholarship. Just as bad money drives out good, athletes using performance-enhancing drugs will ultimately make those who choose not to a minority at the interscholastic level unless educational and testing regulations are stringently implemented and enforced.

Limitations and Future Research

As with many investigations there are limitations. First, we examined the responses of athletic directors of only three state interscholastic associations. Therefore, the results of this study cannot be generalized to a national basis. However, it should be noted that the response rate was 35%, which is above the acceptance rate for online survey research (Anderson and Gansneder, 1995). Second, it can only be assumed that the respondents responded in a truthful and honest fashion. Lastly, the athletic directors that did not participate in the study may have in fact possessed suspicions or beliefs regarding steroid use and testing but simply choose not to disclose it.

Future research may include athletic directors in all 50 state associations regarding their perceptions of steroid use in interscholastic athletics to determine whether the results of this survey can be applied to a greater population. Additional research could further explore the idea regarding the perceived use of steroids by interscholastic athletes as well as others involved in extracurricular high school activities. Finally, given the increased opportunities that exist to continue competition at the intercollegiate and professional levels, a study could deal with the female interscholastic athletes who may be or have taken performance-enhancing drugs such as steroids.

REFERENCES

American College of Sports Medicine. (2004). *The use of anabolic-androgenic steroids in sports.* Retrieved September 5, 2007 from http://www.acsm.org/publications/newsreleases2004/steroids071404.htm.

Anderson, S. E., and Gansneder, B. M. (1995). Using electronic mail surveys and computer monitored data for studying computer mediated communication systems. *Social Science Computer Review, 13*(1), 33-46.

Bahrke, M. S. and Yesalis, C. E. (November, 2002). The future of performance-enhancing substances in sport. The Physician and Sportsmedicine, 30(11), 51-53.

Bhasin, S., Storer, T.W., Berman, N., Callegari, C., Clevenger, B., Phillips, J., Bunnell, T. J., Tricker, R., Shirazi, A., and Casaburi, R. (1996). The effects of supraphysiological doses of testosterone on muscle size and strength in normal men. New England Journal of Medicine, 335(1), 1-7.

Blue Cross Blue Shield. (2003). Blue Cross/Blue Shield says 1.1 Million teens have used performance enhancing sports supplements and drugs. Retrieved on September 24, 2007.from http://www.supplementquality.com/news/ephedra_teens_BCBS.html

Board of Education v. Earls, 2002 U.S. LEXIS 4882.

Centers for Disease Control and Prevention. (May 2004). National youth risk behavior survey: 1991-2003. *Morbidity and Mortality Weekly Report.* Retrieved on October 25, 2007 from http://www.cdc.gov/mmwr/PDF/SS/SS5302.pdf.

Dickerson, J. (2005). *Shooting stars.* Retrieved on December 7, 2007, from http://www.timespublications.com/sept05-feature1.asp

Fainaru-Wada M. (December 19, 2004). Dreams, steroids, death: A ballplayer's downfall. *San Francisco Chronicle*, A1.

Florida High School Athletic Association. (2007). *2007-08 state of Florida/FHSAA anabolic steroid testing program.* Retrieved on December 3, 2007, from http://www.fhsaa.org/compliance/steroid_testing/drug_test_prog_info.pdf

Florida High School Athletic Association. (2007). *Consent of member school to participate in random testing of student-athletes in grades 9-12 for use of anabolic steroids.* Retrieved on December 3, 2007, from http://www.fhsaa.org/compliance/steroid_testing/drug_school_consent_form.pdf

Florida Statutes. (2007). *1006.20 athletics in public K-12 schools.* Retrieved on December 3, 2007, from http://www.leg.state.fl.us/statutes/index.cfm?App_mode=Display_StatuteandURL=Ch1006/ch1006.htm

Grunbaum, J. A, Kann. L, Kinchen, S. A, Ross, J., Hawkins, J., Lowry, R., Harris, W.A., McManus, T., Chyen, D., and Collins, J. (2004).Youth risk behavior surveillance: United States - 2003. *Morbidity and Mortality Weekly Reports Surveillance Summaries, 53,* 1 –96.

Heckman, D. (2003). The evolution of drug testing of interscholastic athletes. *Villanova Sports and Entertainment Law Journal, 9,* 209-228.

International Herald Tribune. (2007). *Doping: China cracking down on the drug industry: Drugs.* Retrieved on December 3, 2007, from http://www.iht.com/articles/2007/11/08/sports/DRUGS.php#end_main

Jacobs, J. B. and Samuels, B. (1994). The drug testing project in international sports: Dilemmas in an expanding regulatory regime. *Hastings International and Comparative Law Review, 18,* 557- 590 .

Johnston, L. D., O'Malley, P. M., Bachman, J. G., and Schulenberg, J. E. (2003). *Monitoring the future: National results on adolescent drug use, overview of key findings.* Retrieved on October 14, 2007 from http://www.monitoringthefuture.org/pubs/monographs/overview2003.pdf.

Justice Talking Radio Transcript. (August 21, 2006). *Does drug testing student athletes deter drug use?* Retrieved on November 1, 2007 from http://www.justicetalking.org/transcripts.pdf.

Kallestad, B. (2005). *Steroid cleanup takes aim at teens.* Retrieved October 23, 2007 from http://www.washtimes.com/national/20050425-122712-5045r.htm.

Latiner, C. (Summer, 2006). Steroids and drug enhancement in sports: The real problem and the real solution. *DePaul Journal of Sports Law and Contemporary Problems, 3,* 192-219.

McDevitt, E. R. (2003). Ergogenic drugs in sports. In: DeLee, J. and Drez, D.(eds.), *Orthopaedic Sports Medicine: Principles and Practice.* 2nd ed. (471 –483). Philadelphia, PA: WB Saunders.

Miller, J. and Wendt, J.T. (2007). Interscholastic athletic directors perceptions of steroid use: A state study. *Journal of Contemporary Athletics, 2*(3), 207-224.

Miller, J., Wendt, J. T. and Seidler, T. (in press). Tackling steroid abuse in interscholastic athletics: Perceptions of athletic directors. *International Journal of Sport Management.*

Moore, D. L. (May 5, 2005). As steroid use doubles, a school fights back: How one high school is educating coaches and students is at the heart of a policy California might adopt this week, *U.S.A. Today,* 1A.

National Federation of State High School Associations. (2003). *Sports medicine: high school drug-testing programs.* Retrieved on November 30, 2007 from www.nfhs.org.

National Institute on Drug Abuse. (2004). *Research report series – Anabolic steroid abuse 1.* Retrieved on December 11, 2007 from http://www.nida.nih.gov/PDF/RRSteroi.pdf.

New Jersey State Interscholastic Athletic Association. (2007). *NJSIAA steroid testing policy.* Retrieved December 3, 2007, from http://www.njsiaa.org/NJSIAA/07steroidmemo.pdf

New Jersey State Interscholastic Athletic Association. (2007). *NJSIAA steroid testing policy: Consent to random testing.* Retrieved December 3, 2007, from http://www.njsiaa.org/NJSIAA/07policyconsent.pdf

New Jersey State Interscholastic Athletic Association. (2007). *NYJSIAA steroid testing policy: Frequently asked questions.* Retrieved December 3, 2007, from http://www.njsiaa.org/NJSIAA/Steroid-FAQ.pdf

New Jersey v. T.L.O., 469 U.S. 325, 338 (1985).
Palmer v. Merluzzi, 689 F. Supp. 400, 412, 415 (D.N.J. 1988).
Paolo, A. M., Bonaminio, G. A., Gibson, C., Patridge, T., and Kallail, K. (2000). Response rate comparisons of e-mail and mail distributed student evaluations. *Teaching and Learning in Medicine, 12 (2),* 81-84.
Patten, M.L. (2000). *Questionnaire research: A practical guide.* Los Angeles, CA: Pyrczak Publishing.
Pells, E. (2007). *States find difficulty imposing high school steroid tests.* Retrieved December 7, 2007, from http://www.southcoasttoday.com/apps/pbcs.dll/article?AID=/20070708/SPORTS/707080377.
Pope, H. G, Kouri, E. M, and Hudson, J. I. (2000). Effects of supraphysiologic doses of testosterone on mood and aggression in normal men: A randomized controlled trial. *Archives of General Psychiatry, 57*(2), 133-140.
Schaill v. Tippecanoe County School Corporation, 864 F.2d 1309 (7th Cir. 1988).
State of New Jersey. (2005). *Executive order #72, acting governor Richard J. Codey.* Retrieved December 3, 2007, from http://www.state.nj.us/infobank/circular/eoc72.htm
Scharrer, G. (2007). *School steroid-testing plan may be posted today.* Retrieved December 7, 2007, from http://www.chron.com/disp/story.mpl/metropolitan/5330838.html.
Shutler, S.E. (Summer, 1996). Random, suspicionless drug testing of high school athletes. *Journal of Criminal Law and Criminology, 86*(4), 1265-1304.
States consider high school steroid testing. (2005). Retrieved September 21, 2007, from http://www.msnbc.msn.com/id/7628183/.
Sturmi, J. E. and Diorio, D. J. (1998). Anabolic agents. *Clinical Sports Medicine, 17,* 261-282.
University Interscholastic League. (2007). *UIL banned substance testing questions and answers.* Retrieved December 3, 2007, from http://www.uil.utexas.edu/athletics/forms/pdf/policy/steroid_testing_faq.pdf
University Interscholastic League. (2007). *UIL parent and student Notification/Agreement form: Illegal steroid use and random steroid testing.* Retrieved December 3, 2007, from http://www.uil.utexas.edu/athletics/forms/pdf/policy/steroid_agreement.pdf.
University Interscholastic League. (2007). *UIL testing protocol.* Retrieved December 3, 2007, from http://www.uil.utexas.edu/athletics/forms/pdf/policy/UIL_testing_protocol.pdf.
Vernonia School District 47J v. Acton , 515 U.S. 646, 115 S. Ct. 2386, 132 L. Ed. 2d 564, 1995 U.S. LEXIS 4275, 63 U.S.L.W. 4653, 9 Fla. L. Weekly Fed. S 229, 95 Cal. Daily Op. Service 4846 (1995).

White House Office of National Drug Control Policy. (2007). *White House drug czar heralds results of New Jersey random student steroid testing.* Retrieved December 3, 2007, from http://www.whitehousedrugpolicy.gov/news/press07/101007.html.

Yamaguchi, R., O'Malley, P.M., and Johnston, L.D. (Winter, 2004). Relationships between school drug searches and student substance use in U.S. Schools. *Educational Evaluation and Policy Analysis, 26*(4), 329-341.

Zirkel, P. A. (2000). Suspicionless searches. *Principal, 79*(5), 57–61.

In: Sports Medicine and Training Tools
Editors: B. Carmichael and A. Mitchell

ISBN: 978-1-61122-827-4
© 2011 Nova Science Publishers, Inc.

Chapter IV

THE IMPORTANCE OF PARENT PHYSICAL ACTIVITY LEVELS AND THEIR EXPECTATIONS FOR THEIR CHILDREN'S HEALTH: A PATH ANALYSIS

Marc Lochbaum*, Tara Stevens, Yen To and Sarah Stevenson
Texas Tech University, USA

ABSTRACT

Rates of childhood obesity are reaching epidemic levels. The purpose of this investigation was to determine if parent behavior and expectations are associated with estimates of their children's leisure time activities and their adult body size. Bandura's (1986) social cognitive theory guided the investigation. Participants were 121 parents of 65 kindergarten and 56 fifth grade students from a midsized rural school district. The majority of parents

---

* Correspondence for this manuscript should be addressed to: Marc Lochbaum, Ph.D. Department of Health, Exercise and Sport Sciences, Texas Tech University, Box 43011. Lubbock, Texas 79409-3011. Email: marc.lochbaum@ttu.edu. 806.742.3371 (phone). 806.742.1688 (fax)

were minorities with a low percentage of parents having obtained degrees beyond a high school diploma. Parents completed measures to assess their physical activity level, their preferences for their children's leisure time activity, estimates of time spent in a variety of leisure time activities, and an estimate of their children's adult body size as an adult. Parents spent very little time in physical activity though their preference was for their children to be active. Path analysis was conducted on a model that described relationships between parents' activity levels and their preferences for their children's activity, parents' activity levels and that of their children, and parents' preferences for their children's physical activity and their children's time spent in physical activity. An association was also posited between parents' preferences for their children's physical activity and their children's body size as an adult. Path analysis goodness of fit indices indicated a good fit (e.g., $SRMR = .02$, $CFI = 1.00$). All associations were in the hypothesized direction. In addition, the greater preference for children to be active was associated with a decrease in estimated body size as an adult by the parents. The percent of variance accounted for (< 10%) in the significant paths do suggest that several important variables were missing in our model. Future research longitudinal research that incorporates more extensive measures of both parents and their children are discussed.

Keywords: social cognitive theory; childhood obesity; adult obesity.

INTRODUCTION

It is far too common to hear parents to say to their children "do as I say, not as I do." Most likely these parents are failing to serve as appropriate role models for their children's behavior, and thus, their development. Social cognitive theory emphasizes the role of models and observational learning in children's development (Bandura, 1986). Social cognitive theory ostensibly supports the importance of actual parent behavior when considering parents' influence on their children's development. It is important to note that Bandura (1986, 2001) has also described individuals as agents in their own behavior. That is, individuals (children) who observe models (their parents) will process the models' behavior and make determinations about the reproduction of the behavior. The determination about reproduction depends upon the context of personal characteristics and considerations of rewards and consequences. This explanation suggests that children do have the capability of avoiding behavior learned through observation, even when the model is a parent.

The American public is now well aware that an obesity epidemic is plaguing the country. Not only are American adults growing larger (U.S. Census Bureau, 2007), but so also are American children (CDC, 2007; Deckelbaum and Williams, 2001). The National Center for Health Statistics (2006) reported that approximately 25 million American children were currently obese or overweight revealing a 300% increase in childhood obesity rates since 1980. Currently, at least 15 states are reported to have at least 26% of their adult population as obese (TFAH, 2007). Even more shocking, 32 states are reported to have 60% of their adult population classified as either overweight or obese (TFAH, 2007) with the majority of these states being in the southwestern region of the country. In addition, it is not surprising to find that the states with the highest rates of obesity are generally the same states with the highest rates of physical inactivity (TFAH, 2007).

The current cost in healthcare and physical and mental well-being is staggering as our society continues to grow predominantly obese. Adult obesity and physical inactivity is linked to numerous health care problems ranging from hypertension, coronary heart disease, diabetes, stroke, and some cancers (CDC, 2006a; Flegal, Carroll, Kuczmarski, and Johnson, 1998; TFAH, 2007). Consequentially, the annual cost of obese and overweight adults to that nation's health care system fluctuates from a low of $69 billion to a high of $117 billion (DHHS, 2003). According to researchers the cost of adult physical inactivity, overweight, and obesity accounts for over 25% of total health care costs in the U.S. (Anderson, Martinson, Crain, Pronk, Whitebird, O'Connor, et al., 2005). For children, ages 6 to 17 years, one study revealed the associated hospital costs of obesity amplified three-fold from a cost of $35 million in 1979 to more than $127 million in 1999 (Wang and Dietz, 2002).

The CDC reported in 2006 that more than 22% of the adult population in the U.S. report not engaging in any physical activity (CDC, 2006b). In addition more than half of adults do not engage in 20 minutes of vigorous activity three times per week, the CDC's recommended level of physical activity. Many have considered that the lack of parents' physical activity is influencing the sedentary lifestyle of their children (Arluk, Branch, Swain, and Dowling, 2003; Fogelholm, Nuutinen, Pasanen, Myöhänen, and Säätelä, 1999; Polley, Spicer, Knight, and Hartley, 2005). Parents are modeling a sedentary lifestyle absent of vigorous activity for their children; however, parents are also showing their preference for their children's physical activity through their increased support of organized sports as 20 to 25 million children participate in organized youth sports each year and an additional 25 in organized public/private school sports (Hutchinson and Ireland, 2003; Tanji, 1991). It is very important to gain an understanding as to whether or not children are more likely to develop physical activity habits based on what they observe their parents doing or based on what they hear their parents saying? Hence, the purpose of our research is to address this question through the evaluation of a path model based on theoretical propositions that posits relationships between parents' levels of physical activity, parents' preferences for their children's physical activity, and estimates of the time the children actually spend engaged in vigorous physical activity.

BACKGROUND OF PRESENT INVESTIGATION

Through social interactions, individuals develop self-perspectives and beliefs that influence their behavioral choices and selection of environments. Although children observe their parents' physical activity levels, this information is routed through their self-perspectives and beliefs. Thus, a bidirectional relationship exists between individuals, their behavior, and the environment to create triadic reciprocal causality (Bandura, 1986). When considering the problem of obesity, children will likely observe the physical activity of a wide variety of individuals; however, children are most frequently exposed to their parents (Moore, Lombardi, White, Campbell, Oliveria, and Ellison, 1991). Also, during the elementary years, parents still provide an important influence on their children's behavior (Coley, 1998; Singer and Miller, 1999). Therefore, one would expect parents to be a model higher in status than the others, which would make it more likely that young children would select to model their parents' behavior. Additionally and critical to social cognitive theory, the frequent exposure children have to their parents would assist in children's ability to recall and reproduce the behavior. Specifically, based on recall and reproduction of observed behaviors, one would expect that children who observe highly active parents will be more active than children who observe their parents being mainly sedentary.

Interestingly, researchers have failed to find a significant relationship between parents' levels of physical activity and that of their children (e.g., Anderssen, Wold, and Torsheim, 2005; Trost, Sallis, Pate, Freedson, Taylor, and Dowda, 2003). Anderssen et al. (2005) conducted a longitudinal study of 557 adolescents across an eight year period. The researchers assessed both the parents and their children's self-reported levels of leisure-time physical activity. The researchers also evaluated the associations between changes in parents' physical activity and the changes in their adolescents' physical activity over the eight year period.

Results did not reveal statistically significant associations and indicated the presence of either weak or non-existent relationships.

Similar to Anderssen and colleagues (2005), Trost et al. (2003) evaluated the physical activity levels of adolescents utilizing a sample of 380 middle and high school students as well as their parents. In addition to assessing physical activity levels of all participants, the authors assessed parental support for physical activity and their children's self-efficacy perceptions related to physical activity participation. These variables were assessed to test a theoretical model positing a relationship between parent physical activity orientation and their children's physical activity that was routed through parental support and self-efficacy for physical activity. The authors reported that the model failed to provide adequate fit to the data, but identified parental support as an important correlate of children's physical activity through its association with self-efficacy in a revised model with path coefficients ranging from 0.17 to 0.24. Thus, the authors did not find parental levels of physical activity to be an important factor in the prediction of children's physical activity, but found parents' capacity to provide motivational support to be important.

In addition to Trost and colleagues (2003), Davison, Cutting, and Birch (2003) reported that parent support of physical activity was associated with children's physical activity. Davison and colleagues utilized a sample of 180 nine-year-old girls and their parents to evaluate the relationship between activity-related parenting strategies and children's physical activity patterns. Significantly higher levels of physical activity were observed in girls who had at least one parent who reported high levels of physical activity support when compared to girls who had no parent providing such support.

The findings suggest that parents' modeling of physically active behavior tends to be much less influential than their support of their children's participation in physical activity concerning their children's physical activity behavior. Social Cognitive Theory's triadic reciprocal causation gives credence to models and observational learning; however, not only does the model influence the viewer but the viewer has the opportunity to evaluate the model. Anderssen et al., (2005) and Trost et al., (2003) both investigated adolescents who likely had opportunities to interact with peers as well as other adults. As a result, these children likely had multiple models from which to choose behavior. Moreover, as children enter into adolescence they tend to be less interested in their parents as their peers begin to gain more influence over their decisions (Biddle, Bank, and Marlin, 1980; Eccles, 1999). The failure to find a relationship between parent physical activity and the physical activity of adolescents could be explained by these issues; however, elementary children typically spend more time with their parents than do adolescents. In addition, children tend to identify with their parents (Peretti and Statum, 1984a, 1984b) more so than with their peers. Hence, parents tend to be more important models than peers for younger children than for adolescents.

Finally, one must consider that although the influence of parents' physical activity on the activity level of their children is questionable, parents' physical activity is likely related to parents' preferences for their children's physical activity. This relationship seems plausible as inconsistency between beliefs and behavior can result in discomfort (Festinger, 1957). Parents who engage in physical activity likely possess some beliefs about the value and importance of such behavior. To not ascribe similar beliefs to the activity levels of their children would be unusual; thus, parents who are physically active likely encourage or support their children in such endeavors.

Purpose and Hypotheses of Present Investigation

The purpose of the present study was to simultaneously evaluate the importance of both parent activity level and parent encouragement of children's physical activity in the prediction of children's time spent in vigorous physical activity as well as to evaluate the role of parent encouragement in the prediction of children's expected body size. A path model was developed that evaluated these relationships. A positive association was hypothesized between parents' level of physical activity and parent preference for their children's physical activity as well as children's time spent in physical activity. Finally, parents' expectations of their children's adult body size, was included in the model to gain insight into the specific problem of obesity. We hypothesized parents' preferences for their children's physical activity would be negatively associated to their estimation of their children's body size as an adult.

METHOD

Participants

Participants were 121 parents of 65 kindergarten and 56 fifth grade students who were attending a rural, yet midsized, school district in the Southwestern United States. The average age of the mothers was 33.16 ($SD = 6.35$) and the average age of the fathers was 35.81 ($SD = 7.83$). The mothers' ethnicity was most frequently described as Hispanic/Latino (56.2%), followed by White (37.2%), Black/African American (1.7%), American Indian/Alaskan Native (.8%), and Asian (.8%). Four (3.3%) of the parents described the mother's ethnicity as other or failed to endorse a category. Similarly, the fathers' ethnicity was most frequently described as Hispanic/Latino (56.2%), followed by White (32.2%), Black/African American (5.0%), and American Indian/Alaskan Native (.8%). Four (3.3%) of the parents described the father's ethnicity as other or failed to endorse a category.

The educational level of both mothers and fathers in the sample was typically less than a bachelor's degree. The majority of the mothers (36.4%) were described as being a high school graduate. The remainder was reported as having some college but no degree (28.9%), less than a high school education (17.4%), a bachelor's degree (10.7%), an associate's degree (5.0%), a master's degree (.8%), and doctoral degree (.8%). Similar to the mothers, the majority of the fathers (39.7%) were described as being a high school graduate. However, in contrast to the mothers, a larger number of fathers were reported as having less than a high school education (28.9%). The remaining fathers were described as having some college but no degree (13.2%), a bachelor's degree (5.8%), an associate's degree (5.0%), a master's degree (1.7%), and doctoral degree (.8%).

Instruments

Parents' Physical Activity. The International Physical Activity Questionnaire (2005 [IPAQ]) Short Form was utilized to evaluate parents' physical activity levels. The IPAQ was developed for use with individuals ranging from 15 to 69 years of age and designed to yield both categorical and continuous estimates of adult physical activity. The IPAQ requested that parents record the number of days during the last seven that they engaged in vigorous physical activity, moderate physical activity, and walking. In addition, they were asked to estimate how much time in hours and minutes that they typically spent doing those types of activities. A final question asked parents how much time they spent on a typical day sitting during the last seven. The volume of activity was computed by weighting each type of activity (i.e., vigorous, moderate, and walking) by its energy requirements which are defined in multiples of the resting metabolic rate or MET. These MET values for each activity were derived from the Ainsworth et al. Compendium (2000). MET values are not calculated for the sitting question as the MET is an estimate of energy expenditure, which is limited in sitting. Instead, the sitting score simply reflects the minutes parents engaged in sitting.

The IPAQ has frequently been utilized to assess adult physical activity (e.g., Al-Hazzaa, 2007; Meriwether, McMahon, Islam, and Steinmann, 2006; Timperio, Salmon, Rosenberg, and Bull, 2004), and the evaluation of the reliability and validity associated with IPAQ scores has extended across countries (e.g., Craig, Marshall, Sjostrom, Bauman, Booth, Ainsworth, et al., 2003; Ekeland, Sepp, Brage, Becker, Jakes, Hennings, and et al., 2006; McFarlane, Lee, Ho, Chan, and Chan, 2006) and special populations (e.g., Faulkner, Cohn, and Remington, 2006). Brown, Trost, Bauman, Mummery, and Owen (2004) found evidence supporting acceptable levels of test-retest reliability for both activity status and sedentary behavior. Craig et al. (2003) also found support for reliability and validity of scores through the assessment of test-retest correlations and concurrent correlation with another measure of activity. These results are consistent with those of the test developers (IPAQ, 2007) who assessed 2,450 adults from 14 countries and reported Spearman's Rho that clustered around .8 for repeat administrations over a three to seven day period and a median rho of .30 with the CSA accelerometer for minutes of vigorous, moderate, walking, and sitting behavior.

Parents' Preferences for Children's Activity. To assess parent preferences for their children's engagement in physical activity, parents were asked to rate the types of after school activities in which they preferred their children to participate in for leisure. Parents rated 10 activities from three domains; vigorous activity (e.g., Working out at a gym at school or other location), cognitive activity (e.g., Reading a book or magazine), and sedentary activity (Watching television); using a scale ranging from 1 "strongly discourage" to 10 "strongly encourage." The subscales were calculated by summing the item scores.

Principal components analysis using Promax rotation was employed to evaluate the presence of the three expected factors. Confirmatory factor analysis was not utilized as the small sample size was not appropriate for the evaluation of a model including more than 10 parameters (see Kline, 1998). A clean factor structure resulted with the three factors accounting for 62.53% of the variance (see Table 1). The first factor was indicated by three items associated with vigorous physical activity, the second factor was indicated by three items associated with cognitive activity, and the third factor was indicated by four items associated with sedentary behavior. Internal consistency estimates of Cronbach's alpha for each subscale were .71, .67, and .74, respectively.

Children's Time Spent in Activity. Children's time spent engaged in physical activity was assessed in a manner parallel to that of parents' preferences for children's activity. Parents were asked to record how much time (i.e., hours and minutes) their children actually spend engaging in the activities identified in the preferences measure during a typical week. Totals in minutes were calculated for each domain; vigorous activity, cognitive activity, and sedentary behavior.

Children's Adult Body Size Expectation. Children's expected adult body size was estimated by their parents through the use of a set of gender specific pictures ranging from an adult of slight build (i.e., 1) to one that is clearly obese (i.e., 9). These pictures were similar to those of Thompson and Gray (1995). With nine body sizes included, parents were asked to circle the image that they believed their child's body will look like as an adult. The researchers then recorded the associated number between one and nine that corresponded to the parents' response.

Table 1. Factor Loadings for Parents' Preference for Children's Activity Measure

Items	Factor		
	Vigorous	Cognitive	Sedentary
Attending specialized activity classes (e.g., gymnastics, karate, ballet, etc.)	.86		
Playing on an organized sports team	.81		
Working out at a gym (at school or other location)	.51		
Reading a book or magazine		.82	
Playing a game outside with friends		.78	
Playing board games (puzzles, checkers, etc.)		.61	
Playing video games			.85
Watching television			.79
Watching videos or movies			.69
Playing on the computer (surfing the internet, etc.)			.66

Procedure

Upon receiving permission from the superintendent and administrative personnel, parent contact information was collected from all kindergarten and fifth grade campuses in a school district located in the Southwest. Parents were mailed a consent form requesting their participation as well as the questionnaire in both Spanish and English. A self-addressed envelope was also included in the mailing for parents to return the forms directly to the researchers. In addition to the mail out, consent forms and questionnaires were distributed from the school several weeks later as a reminder. The return rate was approximately 14%, which reflected the schools' stated response rate for similar information requests.

RESULTS

Descriptive Statistics

Means and standard deviations for each variable are presented in Table 2. Consistent with the research describing the use of the IPAQ, the present scores were extremely skewed with the majority of parents expending limited amounts of energy through vigorous, moderate, or walking activity. Due to concern for restricted range in the IPAQ subscales and this effect on correlational analyses (see Table 3), including path analysis, the total IPAQ score was transformed using logarithmic transformation and a constant of one to bring the smallest value, which was zero, to one (Tabachnick and Fidell, 2001).

Table 2. Means and Standard Deviations for All Variables in Model

Variable	M	SD
Preference		
Vigorous activities	21.77	6.39
Cognitive activities	23.13	4.99
Sedentary activities	15.38	6.44
Time spent		
Vigorous activities	272.36	296.67
Cognitive activities	783.34	779.02
Sedentary activities	885.25	1578.68
Expectation of Body Size	3.36	1.30
Time spent Sitting	249.97	177.99

Note: Values are listed in units of minutes.

A review of the means and standard deviations for the remaining variables indicated that although parents expressed a greater preference for activities that were vigorous physically and cognitive in nature over those activities that were sedentary, parents reported that their children spent the majority of their leisure time engaged in sedentary activities.

In fact, children spent the least amount of time, only about 4.54 hours, engaged in vigorous activity each week. This is in sharp contrast to the 14.75 hours each week they spent involved in sedentary tasks, such as watching television, playing video games, and surfing the Internet. The correlation matrix in Table 3 revealed that parent preferences for their children's activity did not always correlate with their report of how their children actually spent their leisure time. Two of the relationships, one relating to vigorous activity and the other to sedentary activity, were statistically significant; however, the associations were somewhat small. Interestingly, parents' sitting behavior was more strongly related to their activity preferences for their children in comparison to their level of physical activity or IPAQ total score. This was true for the original IPAQ scores as well as for the transformed scores. Parents' sitting behavior was also related to parent estimates of their children's adult body size.

Based on the aforementioned descriptive analyses and concern for the lack of expected correlations between the IPAQ total score, both transformed and not, we decided to proceed with the path analysis using the estimate of parent sitting behavior to represent their activity levels. In addition, we decided to evaluate only vigorous activity in the path analysis as it is the central focus of the paper and tended to be more strongly associated with the expected variables.

Path Analysis

The theoretical model described in Figure 1 was evaluated using LISREL 8.52 (Joreskog and Sorbom, 2002) and the Simplis programming language. Goodness of fit indices were selected based on the recommendations of Hu and Bentler (1999). A two-index presentation strategy that involved an estimate of close to .09 for the maximum likelihood (ML) based standardized root mean squared residual (SRMR) and close to .95 for the ML based comparative fit index (CFI) was employed. Modifications to the path model were not considered as this model was specified based on theory.

Table 3. Correlation Matrix for IPAQ Scales, Parent Preference, and Time Child Spent

Variable	1	2	3	4	5	6	7	8	9	10	11	12
1. Parent Sitting	---											
2. Walk MET	-.15	---										
3. Moderate MET	-.15	.18	---									
4. Vigorous MET	-.16	.38**	.50**	---								
5. Total MET	-.19	.71**	.66**	.88**	---							
6. Transformed TOT	-.16	.48**	.44**	.51**	.63**	---						
Preference												
7. Vigorous	-.26**	.16	.10	.13	.16	.14	---					
8. Cognitive	.09	-.03	.08	-.003	-.01	.07	.43**	---				
9. Sedentary	.21*	.06	-.003	-.10	-.06	-.06	.03	.30**	---			
Time Child Spent												
10. Vigorous	-.003	-.03	.01	-.01	-.003	.14	.28**	.08	-.10	---		
11. Cognitive	.14	-.08	-.02	-.01	-.03	.10	-.06	.16	.17	.20*	---	
12. Sedentary	.08	-.05	-.05	-.08	-.07	.02	-.11	.06	.32**	.09	.74**	---

Note: Multiples of the resting metabolic rate (MET). $*p < .05$, $**p < .01$.

The model fit the data well considering the Hu and Bentler (1999) guidelines ($SRMR$ = .02; CFI = 1.00) as well as other standards for the evaluation of goodness of fit. For example, the estimate of $\chi^2(2)$ was .52, which was not statistically significant (p = .77), and the Tucker Lewis Fit Index or Non Normed Fit Index reached 1.19. The former signals good model to data fit when statistical significance is not achieved and the latter indicates good fit when values are greater than .90 (Tabachnick and Fidell, 2001).

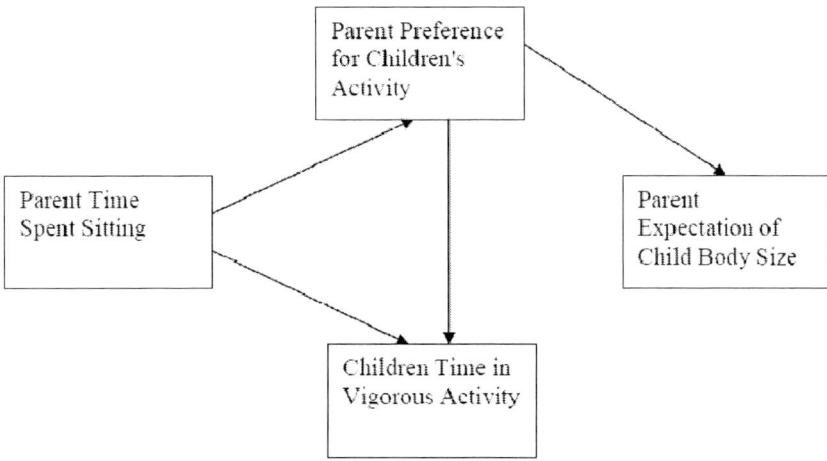

Figure 1. Theoretical model.

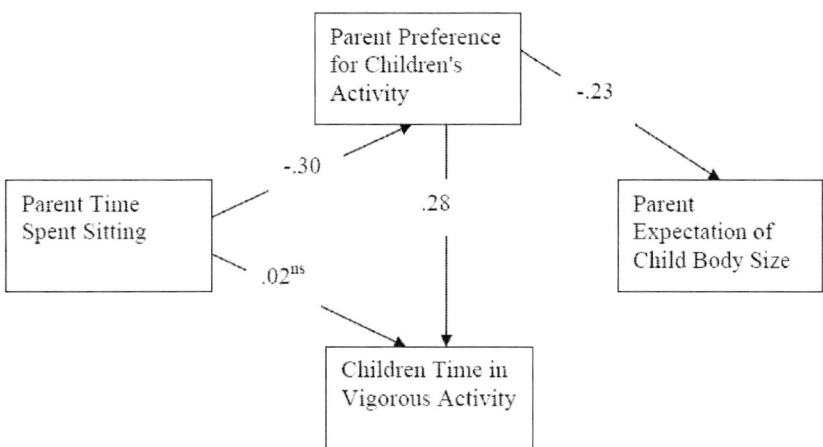

Figure 2. Parameter estimates: Vigorous activity.

All parameter estimates were statistically significant with the exception of the path from parent sitting behavior to children's time spent in vigorous activity (see Figure 2). The remaining variables were related as expected with an increase in sitting behavior associated with a decrease in parent encouragement of their children's vigorous activity and an increase in parent preference for their children's vigorous activity associated with an increase in their children's actual time spent in vigorous activity.

Finally, parents' preference for their children's engagement in vigorous activity was negatively related to their estimates of their children's body size as adults. That is, if parents encouraged the vigorous physical activity of their children, they also expected their children to be smaller in body size once they reach adulthood. Despite the presence of good model to data fit and statistically significant parameters, the amount of variance accounted for in any path was relatively low (less < 10%). The amount of variance in parents' estimates of their children's adult body size accounted for by their preference for their children's vigorous physical activity was 5.5%. Parents' preference for their children's vigorous activity and parents sitting behavior accounted for 7.8% of the variance in children's time spent engaged in vigorous physical activity and parents' sitting behavior accounted for 8.9% of the variance in their preferences for their children's vigorous physical activity.

CONCLUSION

The purpose of the present study was to simultaneously evaluate the importance of both parent activity level and parent encouragement of children's physical activity in the prediction of children's time spent in vigorous physical activity as well as to evaluate the role of parent encouragement in the prediction of children's expected adult body size. A path model was developed and tested to evaluate our purpose. First before integrating our results with theory and past research, the present findings lend support to the growing concern about the shocking number of Americans who live sedentary lifestyles. The level of inactivity of both the parents and children in the present investigation was staggering. Overwhelmingly, participating parents failed to engage in vigorous, moderate, or walking activity. Although this finding is consistent with physical activity trends for adults (Pratt, Macera, and Blanton, 1999), the socioeconomic as well as educational status of parents may have skewed the distribution even further as both are well known factors associated with greater inactivity. The majority of parents in the present sample did not have a college degree. Also, 28.9% of the fathers and 17.4% of mothers reported earning less than a high school diploma.

In sharp contrast to their self-reported physical inactivity, the parents tended to prefer that their children engage in vigorous physical activity, which is encouraging at some level. Fortunately, from Bandura's (1986, 2001) SCT perspective parent encouragement may be more important or at least counteract a poor model in this case a model of physical inactivity. It is important to be reminded that though the parent encouragement that resulted from this preference was associated with higher levels of vigorous physical activity in their children, overall, the children engaged in far more sedentary types of activities than vigorous physical activities. Again, socioeconomic status and or the combination of educational level are factors that could play a role in this discrepancy. Parents might desire that their children be involved in organized sports and work out at the gym; however, they might not have the resources, such as time or money required for transportation or fees, for their children to do so. If parents spend a lot of time at work to compensate for low wages, they likely have less time to support their children's involvement in physical activity. Thus, their encouragement is most likely conveyed verbally rather than through action, which would account for the small amount of variance in children's actual time spent in vigorous physical activity by parent preference for their children's activity.

Parents' preference for their children's vigorous physical activity was more important in the prediction of children's actual time spent in vigorous activity than parents' activity levels, and the parents in the present study did seem to recognize that their preferences in their children's activity would likely influence their children's adult body size. As parents reported providing more encouragement for vigorous physical activity, their estimate of their children's body size as adults declined. Parents do appear to understand the importance of providing support to their children's vigorous activity, which further suggests that other factors tend to prevent children from actually engaging in those types of activities. Therefore, the old adage that indicates children should do as their parents say and not as they do seems to have some validity in the case of physical activity.

The present results support those of Andersson (2005) and Trost et al. (2003). Importantly, the current study extends the lack of an association between parental activity and children's activity to elementary school age children. Although the overall nature of the findings validate concerns for the health of both parents and their children, understanding that parents are able to influence their children's activity levels regardless of their own modeling of physical activity is encouraging. In addition, the results highlight the need for future research. One would expect parent behavior and preferences related to physical activity to have a strong association with the physical activity of children. With researchers consistently finding conflicting results (e.g., Gustafson and Rhodes, 2006), future research is warranted to continue to investigate the influence of peers, school and after school programs, and the media on children's activity levels while also including parental influence in the theoretical framework.

The continued employment of a social cognitive theoretical framework in future research also appears advantageous. Social cognitive theory focuses on individuals as agents in their development (2001), which offers an explanation for children's ability to choose to avoid modeling parent behavior while at the same time heeding their encouragement. In other words, children possess the ability to evaluate the information in their environment and react to it in order to regulate their own behavior. Understanding the apparent self-regulation that appears to be present in the current study should be a focus of future work. "Most of the self-regulation models focus mainly on predicting health behavior, but they offer little operative guidance how to change and maintain it" (Bandura, 2005, p. 248). Bandura (2005) suggested that the cognitive determinants most recently studied in the field can easily be reduced to knowledge of health risks and benefits, self-efficacy or the belief that one can use his/her skills and knowledge to successfully influence health behavior, outcome expectations, health goals, and perceived sociostructural facilitators and impediments. However, no theoretical order is apparent across these cognitive determinants (Bandura, 2005). Furthermore, researchers have predominately studied adults who possess greater control over their choices in activity than do children. The purpose of the present study was to investigate the influence of sociostructural facilitators (i.e., parents) on children's activity, and the goal of future research should be to understand self-regulation in relationship to this influence as self-regulation can be taught to positively impact children's health behavior.

Limitations

Future researchers will also be further guided by the recognition of the present investigation's limitations. First, the sample size was somewhat small and was comprised of individuals living in a rural location in the Southwest. In conjunction with the rural location, the economic opportunities in the area of data collection support mainly unskilled labor. Thus, the socioeconomic status of the majority of participants was somewhat depressed. Low socioeconomic status is a well known factor being associated with lower physical activity patterns. Our measurement of parents' physical activity definitely reflected this association as the self-reported physical activity data was significantly skewed. Researchers in the future should collect data across the range of socioeconomic status that will require purposeful and thoughtful recruitment.

The extremely low parent self-reported physical activity patterns were also problematic in at least on one more way. For instance, these self-reported physical activity patterns were not at all consistent with parent reported beliefs about the importance of physical activity for their children. It could be that for these parents that watching a sporting event is similar to actually participating in that sport though this is hypothetical. For instance, many males played football at some level as adolescents, but as adults few play university level football and almost none play professionally, but the game at both the university and professional levels are very popular television events. It could be that the value of participating in sports such as football is conveyed to children by discussing while viewing the sport on television or attending a local high school game. This behavior of watching a game with one's child or children may be important in predicting their children's activity levels and should be measured (i.e., time spent watching sports together).

Finally, the present study was static in nature. The evaluation of parent influence was at only one time point or cross sectional in nature. To best understand the relationship between parent physical activity and the physical activity of children, several important issues should be addressed. First, researchers should work to follow both the physical activity patterns of parents and their children over time in a more comprehensive manner. For instance, pedometers would greatly assist in gaining a more accurate representation of daily activity. Several psychometrically sound measures of weekly or smaller units of the week exit to provide validation of the pedometer measurement of physical activity. Intervention research would be the last logical step in the research process to examine whether it is the parent actual engagement in physical activity, discussion of the importance of physical activity, or some combination that effects their children's physical activity patterns the most. Though the present research was just an evaluation of a single time point in time, the research has provided provocative results that should excite and guide future research on this topic of extreme urgency.

REFERENCES

Al-Hazzaa, H. M. (2007). Health-enhancing physical activity among Saudi adults using the International Physical Activity Questionnaire (IPAQ). *Public Health Nutrition, 10,* 59-64.

Ainsworth, B. E., Haskell, W. L., Whitt, M. C., Irwin, M. L., Swartz, A. M., Strath, S. J., et al. (2000). Compendium of Physical Activities: An update of activity codes and MET intensities. *Medicine and Science in Sports and Exercise, 32*(9), 498-504.

Anderson, L. H., Martinson, B. C., Crain, A. L., Pronk, N. P., Whitebird, R. R., O'Connor, P. J., and et al. (2005). Health care charges associated with physical inactivity, overweight, and obesity. *Preventing Chronic Disease, 2*(4), 1-12.

Anderssen, N., Wold, B., and Torsheim, T. (2005). Tracking of physical activity in adolescence. *Research Quarterly for Exercise and Sports, 76,* 119-129.

Arluk, S. L., Branch, J. D., Swain, D. P., and Dowling, E. A. (2003). Childhood obesity's relationship to time spent in sedentary behavior. *Military Medicine, 168*(7), 583-586.

Bandura, A. (1986). *Social foundations of thought and action: A social cognitive theory.* Englewood Cliffs, NJ: Prentice Hall.

Bandura, A. (2001). Social cognitive theory: An agentic perspective. *Annual Review of Psychology, 52,* 1–26.

Bandura, A. (2005). The primary of self-regulation in health promotion. *Applied Psychology: An International Review, 54,* 245-254.

Biddle, B. J., Bank, B. J., and Marlin, M. M. (1980). Parental and peer influence on adolescents. *Social Forces, 58*(4), 1057-1079.

Brown, W. J., Trost, S. G., Bauman, A., Mummery, K., and Owen, N. (2004). Test-retest reliability of four physical activity measures used in population surveys. *Journal of Science and Medicine in Sport, 7,* 205-215.

Centers for Disease Control and Prevention (CDC). (2006a). *Overweight and obesity: Home.* Retrieved from U.S. Department of Health and Human Services on September 20, 2006, http://www.cdc.gov/nccdphp/dnpa/obesity/

Centers for Disease Control and Prevention (CDC). (2006b). *Behavioral Risk Factor Surveillance System.* Retrieved from U.S. Department of Health and Human Services on October 25, 2007, http://www.cdc.gov/brfss/

Centers for Disease Control and Prevention (CDC). (2007). *Prevalence of overweight among children and adolescents: United States 2003-2004.* Retrieved from U.S. Department of Health and Human Services on October

23, 2007, http://www.cdc.gov/nchs/products/pubs/pubd/hestats/overweight/overwght_child_03.htm

Coley, R. L. (1998). Children's socialization experiences and functioning in single-men households: The importance of fathers and other men. *Child Development, 69*, 219-230.

Craig, C. L., Marshall, A. L., Sjostrom, M., Bauman, A., Booth, M., Ainsworth, B. E, et al. (2003). International Physical Activity Questionnaire: 12-country reliability and validity. *Medicine and Science in Sports and Exercise, 35*(8), 1381-1395.

Davison, K. K., Cutting, T. M., and Birch, L. L. (2003). Parents' activity-related parenting practices predict girls' physical activity. *Medicine and Science in Sports and Exercise, 35*(9), 1589-1595.

Deckelbaum, R. J., and Williams, C. L. (2001). Childhood obesity: The health issue. *Obesity Research, 9*(4), 239-243.

Ekelund, U., Sepp, H., Brage, S, Becker, W., Jakes, R., Hennings, M., et al. (2006). Criterion-related validity of the last 7-day, short form of the International Physical Activity Questionnaire in Swedish adults. *Public Health Nutrition, 9*, 258-65.

Eccles, J. S. (1999). The development of children ages 6 to 14. *The Future of Children, 9*(2), 30-44.

Faulkner, G., Cohn, T., and Remington, G. (2006). Validation of a physical activity assessment tool for individuals with schizophrenia. *Schizophrenia Research, 82*, 225-231.

Festinger, L. (1957). *A theory of cognitive dissonance*, Evanston, IL: Row and Peterson.

Flegal, K. M., Carroll, M. D., Kuczmarski, R. J., and Johnson, C. L. (1998). Overweight and obesity in the United States: Prevalence and trends, 1960-1994. *International Journal of Obesity, 22*, 39-47.

Fogelholm, M., Nuutinen, O., Pasanen, M., Myöhänen, E., and Säätelä, T. (1999). Parent-child relationship of physical activity patterns and obesity. *International Journal of Obesity, 23*(12), 1262-1268.

Hutchinson, M. R., and Ireland, M. L. (2003). Overuse and throwing injuries in the skeletally immature athlete. *Instructional Course Lectures, 52*, 25-36.

Joreskog, K., and Sorbom, D. (2002). *LISREL 8.52*. Scientific Software International, Inc.

Gustafson, S. L., and Rhodes, R. E. (2006). Parental correlates of physical activity in children and early adolescents. Sports Medicine, 36, 79-97.

U.S. Department of Health and Human Services (DHHS). (2003). Prevention makes common "cents." Retrieved from U.S. Department of Health and Human Services on October 23, 2007, http://healthproject.us/documents/Centscondensed.pdf

Hu, L. T., and Bentler, P. M. (1999). Cutoff criteria for fit indexes in covariance structure analysis: Conventional criteria versus new alternatives. Structural Equation Modeling, 6, 1-55.

International Physical Activity Questionnaire (IPAQ). (2007). *Reliability and validity study.* Retrieved from The International Physical Activity Questionnaire Homepage on May 31, 2007, http://www.ipaq.ki.se/IPAQ.asp?mnu_sel=GGDandpg_sel=JJG.

Kline, R. B. (1998). *Principles and practice of structural equation modeling.* New York: Guilford.

McFarlane, D. J., Lee, C. C., Ho, E. Y., Chan, K. L., and Chan, D. (2006). Convergent validity of six methods to assess physical activity in daily life. *Journal of Applied Physiology, 101,* 1328-1334.

Meriwether, R., McMahon, P., Islam, N., and Steinmann, W. (2006). Physical activity assessment validation of a clinical assessment tool. *American Journal of Preventative Medicine, 31*(6), 484-491.

Moore, L. L., Lombardi, D. A., White, M. J., Campbell, J. L., Oliveria, S. A., and Ellison, R. C. (1991). Influence of parents' physical activity levels on activity levels of young children. *Pediatrics, 118*(2), 215-219.

National Center for Health Statistics (NCHS). (2007). *Obesity still a major problem.* Retrieved from Centers for Disease Control and Prevention and U.S. Department of Health and Human Services on October 23, 2007, http://www.cdc.gov/nchs/pressroom/06facts/obesity03_04.htm.

Polley, D. C., Spicer, M. T., Knight, A. P., and Hartley, B. L. (2005). Intrafamilial correlates of overweight and obesity in African-American and Native-American grandparents, parents, and children in rural Oklahoma. *Journal of the American Dietetic Association, 105*(2), 262-265.

Peretti, P., and Statum, J. (1984a). Authoritarian paternal attitude inter-generational transmission. *Pediatrics International, 26*(4), 534-538.

Peretti, P., and Statum, J. (1984b). Farther-son inter-generational transmission of authoritarian paternal attitudes. *Social behavior and Personality: An International Journal, 12,* 85-89.

Pratt, M., Macera. C. A., and Blanton, C. (1999). Levels of physical activity and inactivity in children and adults in the United States: current evidence and research issues. *Medicine and Science in Sports and Exercise, 31*(11) Supp., S526-S533.

Singer, M. I., and Miller, D. B. (1999). Contributors to violent behavior among elementary and middle school children. *Pediatrics, 104*(4), 878-884.

Tabachnick, B., and Fidell, L. (2001). *Using multivariate statistics* (4th ed). Boston, MA: Allyn and Bacon.

Tanji, J. L. (1991). The preparticipation physical examination for sports. *American Family Physician, 42*(2), 397-402.

Trust for America's Health (TFAH). (2007). *F as in fat: How obesity policies are failing in America.* Retrieved from The Trust for America's Health on October 23, 2007, http://healthyamericans.org/reports/obesity2006/Obesity2006Report.pdf

Thompson, M. A., and Gray, J. J. (1995). Development and validation of a new body assessment scale. *Journal of Body Assessment, 64,* 263.

Timperio, A., Salmon, J., Rosenberg, M., and Bull, F. C. (2004). Do logbooks influence recall of physical activity in validation studies? *Medicine and Science in Sports and Exercise, 36*(7), 1181-1186.

Trost, S. G., Sallis, J. F., Pate, R. R., Freedson, P. S., Taylor, W. C., and Dowda, M. (2003). Evaluating a model of parental influence on youth physical activity. *American Journal of Preventative Medicine, 25*(4), 277-282.

U. S. Census Bureau (2007). *Statistical abstract of the United States-2007 Release.* Retrieved from U.S. Census Bureau on October 23, 2007, http://www.census.gov/prod/www/statistical-abstract.html.

Wang, G., and Dietz, W. H. (2002). Economic burden of obesity in youths aged 6 to 17 years: 1979-1999. *Pediatrics, 109*(5), 81-86.

In: Sports Medicine and Training Tools
Editors: B. Carmichael and A. Mitchell

ISBN: 978-1-61122-827-4
© 2011 Nova Science Publishers, Inc.

Chapter V

BIOENERGETICAL ASSESSMENT AND TRAINING CONTROL AS USEFUL TOOLS TO IMPROVE PERFORMANCE IN CYCLIC SPORTS

Ricardo Fernandes[*], *Eduardo Oliveira, and Paulo Colaço*
University of Porto, Faculty of Sport, CIFI^{2}D, Portugal

ABSTRACT

Training control and evaluation of athletes are currently fundamental tools to increase the efficiency of the training process. Thus, coaches and their collaborators often implement a set of tasks that allow evaluating the level of development of the athletes' performance determinant factors as well as the result and adequacy of the training exercises and programs.

Due to their characteristics (individual, cyclic, closed and combined), several sport modalities, including running, swimming, cycling and rowing, are more prone to be evaluated. From the several determinants of the specific performance of these athletes, the bioenergetical and biomechanical factors are recognizably important and, therefore, focus of attention.

The purpose of the present chapter is to present recent data regarding bioenergetical assessment of performance in cyclic sports, giving more

---

[*] ricfer@fade.up.pt

emphasis to running and swimming. The bioenergetical studies presented focus on the characterization of the capacity and power of the two larger body energy systems (the aerobic and the anaerobic ones) through the assessment of well-known physiological parameters like the anaerobic threshold, the maximal oxygen uptake (and the corresponding velocities) and the maximal blood lactate concentrations. Complementarily, recently proposed tests are also presented (e.g. critical velocity).

We hope that the presented results could be well accepted and usefull to athletes, coaches and scientists in their training control programs, helping them to increase the training efficiency and even contributing to predict performance.

Key Words: Training control, athletes evaluation, advice, physiology

1. CONCEPTUALIZATION

Some of the main tasks of coaches and sport scientists are the training control and evaluation of athletes, which have been considered fundamental tools to increase the efficiency of the training process and also to predict performance. Training control and evaluation of athletes are defined as a set of tasks that allow the evaluation of the results and adequacy of the exercise training and programs as well as the level of development of the determinant factors of performance.

Sport modalities like running, swimming, cycling and rowing, being individual, continuous, cyclic, closed and combined modalities, are more suitable for evaluation than team sports. Running and swimming have been along the years the primary areas of research in Sport Sciences, being published technical and scientific experimental studies since the 1930s (Billat, 1998). Scientific studies of rowing and cycling have more constantly appeared since the 1970s. Due to the high influence of external factors (e.g. wind, water conditions and temperature) that may influence the rowing and cycling tests results when conducted in normal competition conditions, experimental protocols have been conducted manly in laboratory conditions (Lucía et al., 2001; Maestu et al., 2005).

As the enhancing of athletes' performance can no longer be obtained only by the increasing of training volume and by the use of non specific methodologies (Olbrecht, 2000) more objective and specific training sets are required to improve the quality of the training process. Therefore, the importance of the knowledge on performance determinant factors, performance diagnosis methods, and training evaluation and control, is rising in the last two decades.

Following Cazorla (1984), the main aim of the specialists in sports testing is to develop, for each athlete (independently of age or proficiency level), methods to assess his/her motor capacities in order to better understand and develop his/her motor background. Moreover, sports testing should be divided in two complementary activities - the control of training loads and the evaluation of the athletes' evolution - keeping in mind that it should have a close interplay between these two items.

There are several reasons why sport testing is vital for increasing athletes' performance (Pyke, 2000): (i) it establish the individual's strengths and weaknesses; (ii) it allows to monitor progress, controlling the effectiveness of the prescribed training program; (iii) it provides feedback of specific test scores, being an incentive for the athletes to improve in a particular area; (iv) it can educate coaches and athletes by providing them with a better understanding of the demands of the sport and the attributes required to be successful; (v) it allows prediction of the performance potential through the identification of individuals more suitable for a specific sport modality. We include the illness, injury and overtraining prevention in the period leading up to the competition, which is often seen as fundamental in the training process.

The first task to accomplish when constructing a testing program is to analyze the sport modality and to define which are its performance influencing factors (Cazorla, 1984). Figure 1 illustrates an example of some requirements for competitive running, swimming, cycling and rowing. As can be observed, bioenergetical, biomechanical and psychological factors assume a direct influence and genetic and contextual factors an indirect influence on athletes' performance. The fact that this diagram is referring to individual, cyclic and closed sport modalities somehow reduces the number of variables to consider and therefore the internal variability spectrum. Complementarily, it is important to notice that each group of parameters is closed related with the others, having a strong reciprocal influence.

Although no attempts had been established to estimate the importance of each factor of the several performance determinants presented in Figure 1, it seems logical that bioenergetical parameters are among the principal determinants. To evaluate the above-referred parameters there are a number of criteria that need to be considered, namely that the fact that tests should be relevant (for the athlete's sport), specific (simulating the competition conditions), practical (concerning the location and the availability of subjects), valid (measuring what it claims to measure) and accurate (when compared to a criterion method).

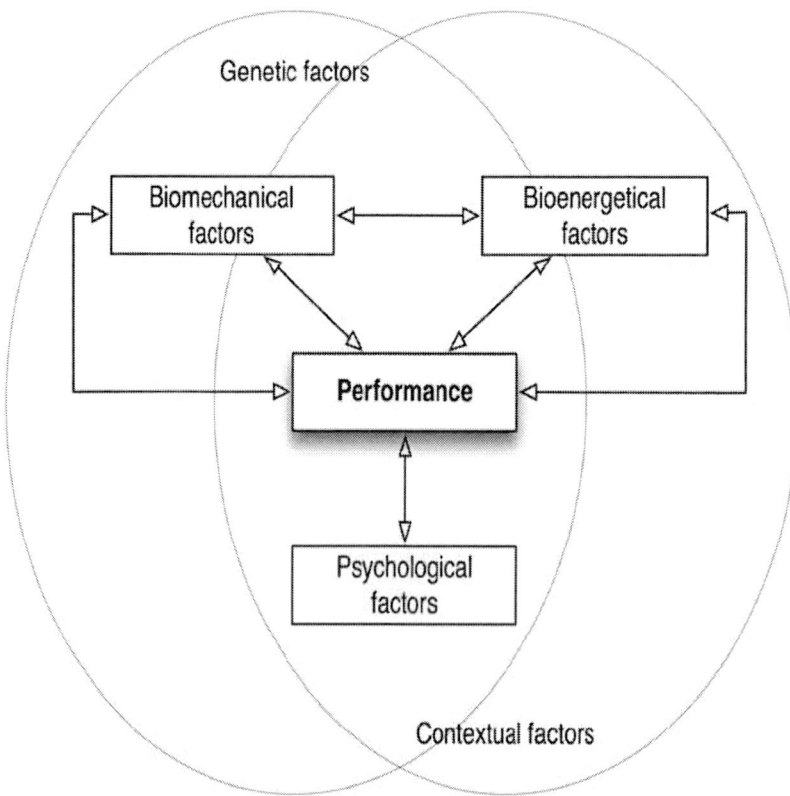

Figure 1. Determinant performance factors in cyclic sports (adapted from Fernandes et al., 2008a).

Considering that running, swimming, cycling and rowing are modalities in which bioenergetical factors assume a fundamental role on performance, the main propose of the present chapter is to present recent data obtained in experimental protocols. It is expected that it could be usefull and applicable by coaches and scientists in their training control programs, helping them to increase the training efficiency and even to explain future performance. In the following sections it will be presented some data more centered in running and swimming, focusing in the characterization of the capacity and power of the aerobic and the anaerobic energy systems through the assessment of well known physiological parameters. In a future paper, some biomechanical studies will be also shown, reporting on movement analysis through bi/three-dimensional kinematics, electromyography and dynamometry.

2. BIOENERGETICAL STUDIES

2.1. Introduction

Performance determinants related to athlete's bioenegetics have been frequently studied. Its main purpose is to determine the bioenergetical profile and to follow the corresponding physiological changes due to the training process. Inclusively, it is well accepted that the increasing development of a series of tests is due at least in some extent to the great interest in the correct establishment of training volumes and intensities, as well as in the selection of the ideal work/rest ratios (Troup, 1995). Thus, the present work show some valid and well accepted tests conducted by our group that allow coaches and scientists to dispose objective and pertinent data related to the aerobic and anaerobic body energy systems. Due to the characteristics of the majority of the events in running, swimming, cycling and rowing, the energetic contribution of high-energy phosphates wasnot taken into account along the text.

2.2. Aerobic System

Our studies have been supported in the proposals of Mader et al. (1976) and Heck et al. (1985), namely when it was estimated the maximal lactate steady-state (Maxlass), trying to achieve an objective indicator to be used in the training field. However, the Maxlass concept is dificult to operate in the training process due to the high number of sessions needed to assess it. In this sense, to determine the correct training intensities in order to develop the aerobic capacity, the anaerobic threshold (AnT) seems to be an accurately way to achieve the Maxlass (Heck et al., 1985; Jones and Doust, 1998). A widely known field procedure to assess AnT is to use the blood lactate concentration ([La^-]) values corresponding to such exercise load (Heck et al., 1985; Svedhal & MacIntosh, 2003). These concentrations reflect the generation/removal ratio of body metabolic turnover.

The AnT can be determined using several protocols (cf. Svedhal & MacIntosh, 2003). Bearing in mind some specific limitations such as the athlete's age (Santos e Ascenção, 1999), accumulated training and training characteristics (Esteve-Lanao et al., 2005), we have been using the step test (Heck et al., 1985) to assess the running velocity corresponding to 4 mmol/l of [La^-] (v4), a well-accepted valid indicator for AnT determination regardless ateletes specific characteristics. In Atheletics (middle-long distance running), this test is composed by 4 x 2000 m (velocity of 4.2-5.8 m/s according with the athlete's level), increments of 0.4 m/s and 1 min of interval between each step (for capillary blood collection). Our experience with the use of AnT has been very useful considering the feedbacks reported by coaches and athletes during the training advisment. One of the most relevant results obtained was the high correlation values between AnT and performance for different running events (Table 1).

Table 1. Correlation values obtained between different middle and long distance running events and anaerobic threshold (adapted from Colaço, 2007)

Event (m)	Subjects (gender/age in years)	Velocity (m/s)	Correlation ($p < 0.05$)
800	12 males (18.6±0.5)	6.76±0.20	r=0.77
1500	20 males (25.9±2.5)	6.32±0.25	r=0.87
5000	20 males (29.0±4.5)	5.79±0.44	r=0.89
Half Marathon (21097)	20 males (28.6±3.7)	5.17±0.46	r=0.95

The results from this table suggest that the AnT can be considered an interesting performance predictor particularly in long distances, which is in accordance with several authors (e.g. Roecker et al., 1998; Papadopoulos et al., 2003). The data also confirm that AnT can be extremely useful even in middle distances, following the proposals of Duffield et al. (2005) and Spencer & Gastin (2001) for the 800 m and 1500 m events, respectively. This fact is more relevant when velocity at AnT is similar to the velocity obtained in competition as in Half Marathon (Figure 2).

In swimming, due to the mechanical constraints imposed by the aquatic environment, it is common to assess AnT through simple non-invasive tests. From those, we would like to stand out the 30 min continuous test - T30 (Olbrecht et al., 1985) and the critical velocity test (Wakayoshi et al., 1992), which are valid and well accepted by coaches and scientists.

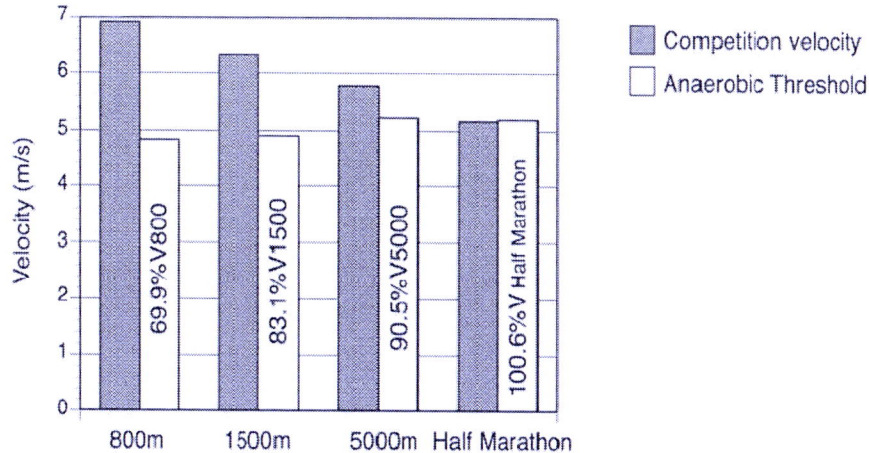

Figure 2. Percentage of v4 values relatively to competition velocity for each middle and long distance event (n = 80; 20 athletes/event). Adapted from Colaço (2007).

Fernandes and Vilas-Boas (1999) observed high relationships between T30 and v4 (r = 0.86, p < 0.01), as well as between critical velocity and v4 (r = 0.82, p < 0.01), being v4 assessed by Mader's two-speed test (Mader et al., 1976). Other works of our group highlighted the relevance of the critical velocity test to training control and evaluation of swimmers of several ages, being easily conducted in a training session (cf. Vilas-Boas et al., 1997; Fernandes et al., 2000; Soares et al., 2003). Examples of critical velocities in age-group to senior swimmers are given in Table 2 (all values were different between genders).

Table 2. Mean plus SD of critical velocity (m/s) for male and female age-group swimmers (adapted from Soares et al., 2003)

	Infant (50 and 400 m)	Juvenile (100 and 800/1500 m)	Junior (100 and 800/1500 m)	Senior (50 and 800/1500 m)
Female	1.10±0.07	1.23±0.05	1.29±0.05	1.34±0.05
Male	1.18±0.08	1.32±0.06	1.36±0.04	1.38±0.07

However, when it is required a more "physiological" approach of the AnT phenomena, a 7 x 200 m intermittent incremental protocol is used (Pyne et al., 2000; Cardoso et al., 2003), in which it is possible to identify the non-linear rise of [La⁻] (Figure 3). This methodology allows us to dispose higher number of [La⁻

]/velocity points which help us to better determine the [La⁻] correspondent to the AnT. Thus, we obtain a better individualization of the AnT (IndAnT) value when comparing to the Mader's two-speed test.

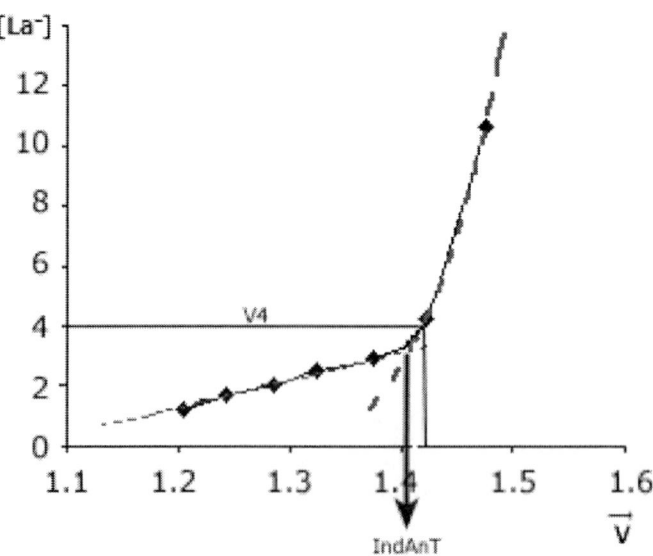

Figure 3. Individual blood lactate concentrations/velocity curve in the incremental test for VO_2max determination. Individual AnT (IndAnT) assessment is represented by the interception of a rectilinear and an exponential line (v4 is also marked). Adapted from Fernandes et al. (2005).

In this figure, it can be observed that the individual [La⁻] values corresponding to AnT are, approximately, 3 mmol/l, lower than the 4 mmol/l value traditionally used. As observed in Santos and Ascensão (1999), in running, this individual value might also achieve higher values than 4 mmol/l. It is likely that the high inter-subject variability of the [La⁻] corresponding to AnT in swimming (Urhausen et al., 1993), as well as the sports specificity of AnT (Beneke and Duvillard, 1996) can contribute to explain this possible diference. Other studies of our group corroborate the example of Figure 3, referring a mean value of 2.99 ± 0.80 mmol/l (Morais et al., 2006) and 2.59 ± 0.97 mmol/l (Fernandes et al., 2008b) for the [La⁻] at AnT.

The blood lactate concentration of 4 mmol/l is also a common reference in rowing, being described that the oxygen consumption, power (W) and velocity at that [La⁻] is closely related to the 2000 m ergometer performance time (Ingham et al., 2002; Womack et al., 1996). However, Beneke (1995) and Jurimae et al. (2001) found values lower than 4 mmol/l for AnT: 3.0 ± 0.6 and 3.7 ± 0.6, respectively. Complementarily, Boiirgois and Vrijens (1998) stated that using fixed or individual lactate threshold values measured on a rowing ergometer as guidelines for training intensity must be viewed with caution because they do not exactly mirror the blood lactate at steady-state for rowers, suggesting the necessity of higher specificity of testing protocols.

Being cycling a long-duration sport, it requires participants to possess high AnT (Lucía et al., 2001). Regarding the metabolic methodologies that can be used to determine the AnT, some authors chosen protocols (4 min increments) to determine the exercise intensity eliciting a blood level of 4 mmol/L (Padilla et al., 1999) or the IndAnT (Fernández-García et al., 2000). Our group has some experience in determining AnT in professional cyclists, namely by conducting an open road intermittent incremental protocol (4 steps of 5 min, with increments of 1.39 m/s). In Table 3 it is possible to observe the values for the heart rate and [La$^-$] for each step of the protocol (n = 14). The mean and SD value for the v4 was 11.32 ± 1.05 m/s.

Table 3. Mean plus SD of heart rate and (beats/min) and blood lactate concentrations in a cycling incremental intermittent protocol (Colaço et al., unpublished data)

	1st step (9.72 m/s)	2nd step (11.11 m/s)	3rd step (12.50 m/s)	4th step (13.88 m/s)
Heart rate (beats/min)	141.2±14.2	158.6±14.3	172.7±8.0	179.4±8.7
Blood lactate concentrations (mmol/l)	1.9±0.6	4.1±2.2	6.0±2.5	7.6±2.6

The [La$^-$]/velocity values referred in the above paragraphs also allow to monitor the exercise increase after the AnT intensity. Data show that, for intensities above the AnT, the increase [La$^-$] rate can be exponential, changing the former linear raising. This fact is more evident in middle distance efforts, in which the exercise intensity is higher. As we can see in Figure 4, the increase [La$^-$] rate is individualized, being different between athletes. This phenomena needs to be regarded as an important factor to be considered (and improved) during the practice. In this sense, the athlete needs a well developed AnT, but also a lower increase [La$^-$] rate for higher exercise intensities.

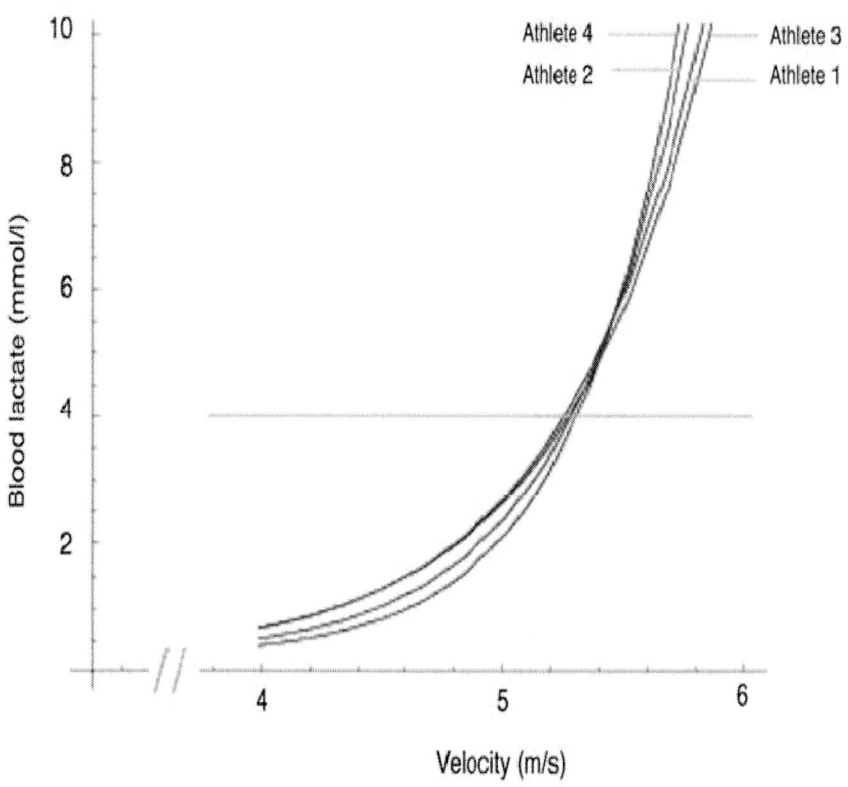

Figure 4. Increase of blood lactate concentration rate in four runners (adapted from Pedro, 2006).

It is possible to observe that the athletes with a better running AnT have a higher increase [La⁻] rate after v4, which is a finding not commonly expected (Pedro, 2006).

In this sense, choosing the correct training volumes for certain specific intensities, it is possible and advisable to adapt the training process in order to combine a well developed AnT and a lower increase [La⁻] rate for higher running velocity. This procedure has been carried out by some of the best coaches (e.g. Canova, 2004), accepting that a well-established physiological adaptation to higher intensities (e.g. 7 mmol/L) lead to a more easily and stable running.

In swimming the increase [La⁻] rate is also studied by us, represented as the slope of the line obtained between 2 steps. In Figure 5, it is possible to observe an example of two [La⁻]/velocity curves (conducted in different moments of the training season) for the same swimmer. We can observe a significant development in the anaerobic component, probably due to the use of more specific training methods recruiting other energy pathways.

Our experiments have been showing the importance of the "increase [La⁻] rate" concept and can justify the reason why some athletes with a lower AnT can performe better in comparison with others. Thus, in Figure 6, it is possible to observe that the athlete #1, presenting a lower developed AnT, has a lower increase [La⁻] rate (defined by a lower slope), which allows him to achieve a better result in Half Marathon compared with other runners (the higher increase [La⁻] rate after the AnT can make them less competitive).

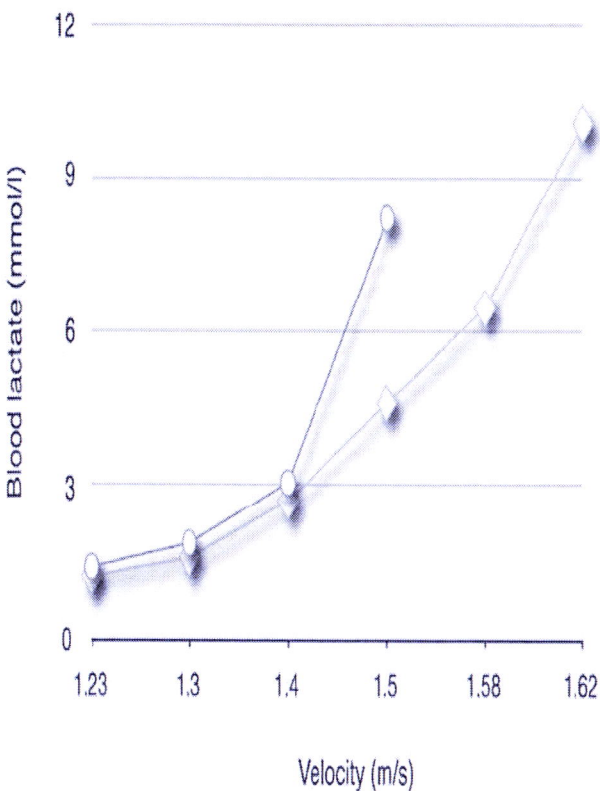

Figure 5. Example of two blood lactate concentrations/velocity curves for the same swimmer conducted in the different moments of the season (Fernandes et al, unpublished data).

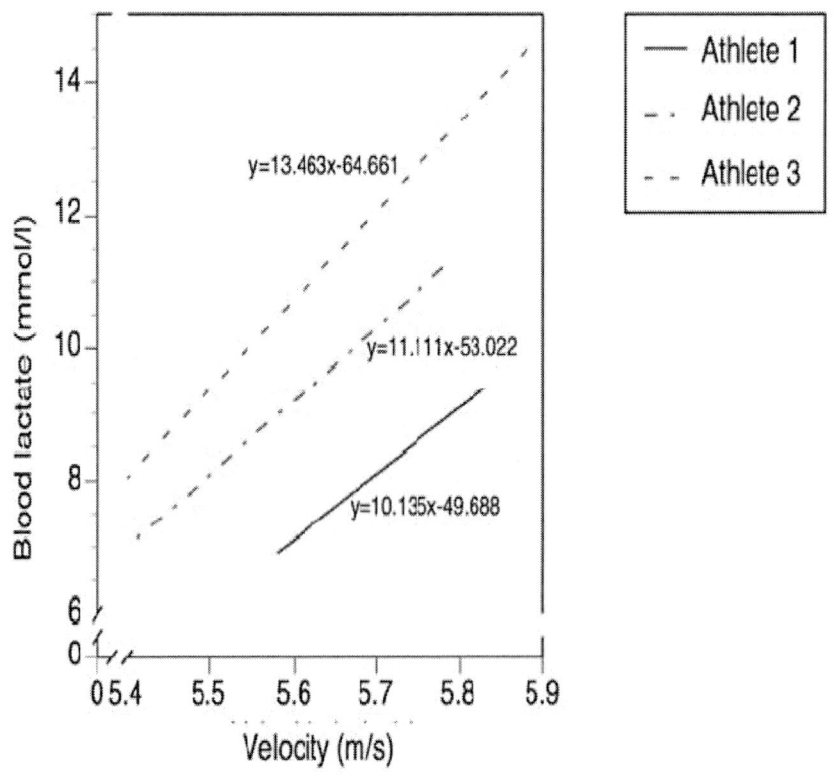

Figure 6. Lines and equations illustrating the increase of blood lactate concentrations rate obtained for three runners in the two last steps of an anaerobic threshold test (adapted from Colaço, 2007).

Additionally, according with data from our group (Pedro, 2006), it is possible to find higher correlation between the 5000 m distance and the velocity corresponding to 6 mmol/L and 7 mmol/L ($r = 0.91$, $p < 0.01$) than for v4, which reinforces the importance of increase [La$^-$] rate after the AnT for middle distance runners. Following the same testing procedure, increase [La$^-$] rate was also evaluated in different moments of the season, which can be fundamental to understand the athlete's progression and to find some eventual evolution problems. It is important to underline that the training adaptations should be conducted in order to improve the AnT, or, in some moments of the season (e.g. the pre-competitive period), to maintain its level of development but also to promote the increase [La$^-$] rate for higher exercise intensities (Figure 7).

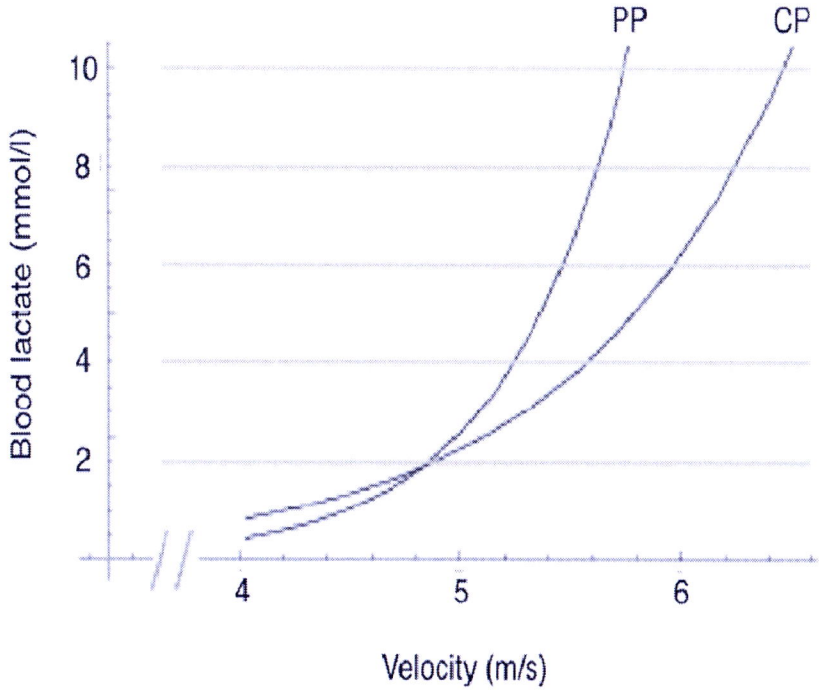

Figure 7. Blood lactate concentration curves corresponded to the preparatory period (PP) and Competitive Period (CP) of a runner (adapted from Pedro, 2006).

From Figure 7 it is possible to refer that, during a season, the athlete should improve the AnT but the improvements corresponding to higher [La⁻] values can be superior. These results suggest that the use of more specific training (as intensive interval training), conducted at higher exercise intensities (e.g. near or at VO2max), can be responsible for the reported improvements. Monitoring these changes can be very useful to readjust the training prescription in a more accurate way. In this regard, we suggest organizing the training process considering different bioenergetical training zones and control possible changes during the season (cf. Olbrecht, 2000).

Considering the establishment of different training zones, we have been studying changes associated to [La⁻]/velocity curves during the season, determining adjacent areas in different [La⁻] intervals and corresponding running velocity, which allows the comparison changes for each athlete during the season (Figure 8). Notice that the higher the area between two [La⁻] values most prepared the athlete is to perform at those intensities.

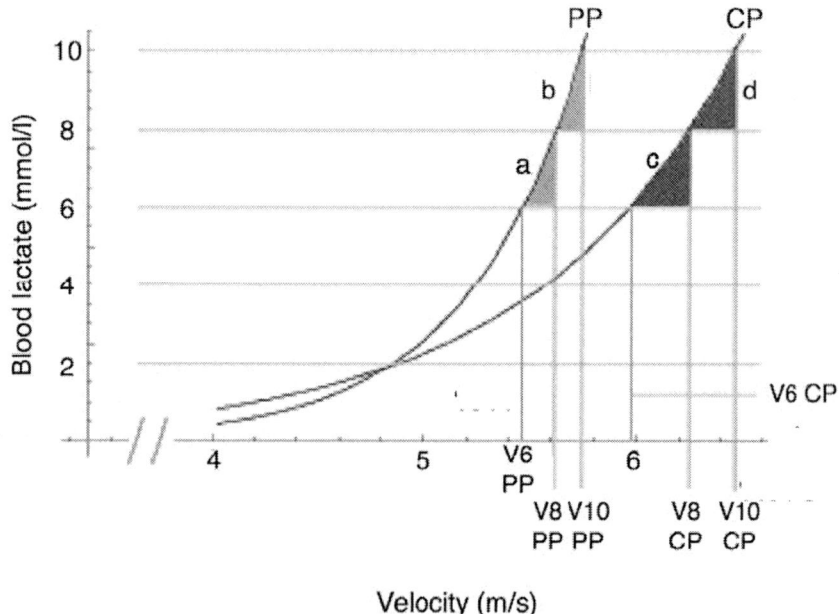

Figure 8. Representation of adjacent areas of blood lactate concentration curves in function of the running velocity, for Preparatory Period (PP - a and b areas) and Competitive Period (CP - c and d areas). Adapted from Pedro (2006).

The oxygen uptake kinetics should also be taken into consideration when evaluating the athletes. Although it is well-known that the methodological procedures to assess VO_2 during exercise are easier to implement in ergometers, some studies of our group were conducted in specific competition conditions. Using the above-referred 7 x 200 m incremental protocol, the VO_2max values for front crawl swimming and its corresponding velocities were assessed in a 25 m swimming pool. The results were 52.1 ± 6.5 ml/kg/min and 1.16 ± 0.10 m/s, 69.9 ± 9.3 ml/kg/min and 1.40 ± 0.06 m/s, and 71.7 ± 6.1 ml/kg/min and 1.45 ± 0.05 m/s, respectively for recreational, competitive and elite male level swimmers (Fernandes et al., 2006a; Fernandes et al., 2008b). At the minimum velocity of VO_2max (vVO_2max), the [La$^-$] were between 8-9 mmol/l and heart rate values between 180-190 b/min, which is in accordance with the specialized literature.

Therafter, we find very interesting to study the swimmer's ability to sustain the vVO_2max intensities, i.e., the swimming intensities that elicit their maximal aerobic power. So, recently, we started focusing in the determination of the time of exercise to exhaustion at vVO_2max (TLim-vVO_2max). This concept has arisen in the last years, seeming to be a very interesting matter for assessing various aspects of performance and training of endurance athletes (Billat et al., 1994). The first studies (e.g. Billat et al., 1996) that assessed TLim-vVO_2max in swimming were conducted using front crawl in swimming flume, not in specific training and competition conditions. As it is accepted that performing in a flume could bring some mechanical constraints, our TLim-vVO_2max related studies were always conducted in a swimming pool. We find a low inter-individual variability in TLim-vVO_2max values, ranging from 215 s in elite swimmers (Fernandes et al., 2008b) to 325 s in low level swimmers (Fernandes et al., 2003a), which are in accordance with the data obtained by Billat et al. (1996) and Demarie et al. (2001) for flume swimming. Those results suggest a lower variation of this parameter in swimming, compared with the results presented for other sports by Billat et al. (1994), namely treadmill running (range 4-11 min). This fact advocate coaches and swimmers to use lower duration of training sets when aiming to develop aerobic power: approximately 5 min in a continuous effort or until 10 min if intermittent training series are used. Moreover, no differences were observed in front crawl TLim-vVO_2max values between genders (Fernandes et al., 2005b), as well as between swimming strokes (Fernandes et al., 2006b), pointing out that the phenomenon is similar in male and female swimmers as well as in all four strokes. In Figure 9 it is represented a typical example of the VO_2 pattern during the TLim-vVO_2max test.

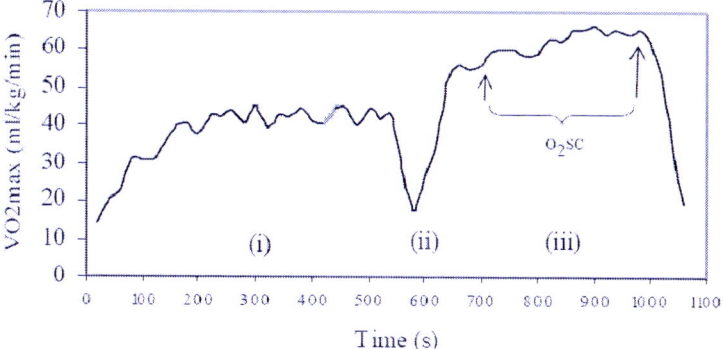

Figure 9. A typical example of the VO_2 pattern during the swimming TLim-vVO_2max test. (i) warm-up; (ii) 20 s rest for capillary blood collection and (iii) maintenance of swimming vVO_2max until exhaustion. The arrows delimit the period where the O_2 slow component was calculated (Fernandes et al., unpublished data).

As it can be depicted from Figure 9, after the fast rise of the VO_2 in the beginning of exercise (just following the cardiodynamic component in the first seconds of exercise), a secondary slower phase of VO_2 kinetics can be observed. This phenomenon, denominated oxygen slow component (O_2SC), seems to contradict the traditional idea of a systematic appearance of a VO_2 plateau after the fast VO_2 kinetics phase in heavy exercise. This fact corroborates the previous studies performed in cycling and running that stated that exercise at metabolic rates above the AnT, i. e., heavy or severe intensity domains, evidences a slowly-developing component of the VO_2 kinetics that is superimposed upon the rapid increase of $\dot{V}O_2$ initiated at exercise onset (Bearden and Moffatt, 2000).

In our studies, O_2SC was assessed as the difference between the last VO_2 measurement of the TLim-vVO_2max test and the last measurement of the second min (Koppo and Bouckaert, 2001) or the third min of exercise (Demarie et al., 2001), being observed amplitudes of 279.0±195.2 ml/min in recreational swimmers (Fernandes et al., 2003a) and 274.1±152.8 in competitive swimmers (Fernandes et al., 2003b) that are in agreement with the Demarie et al. (2001) reports for pentathletes performing in swimming flume. These values seem to be lower than those for running and cycling (Billat et al., 1998), which could be justified by the chosen high exercise intensity and the specificity of this modality. Additionally, in the swimming studies above referred, it were obtained positive relationships between TLim-vVO_2max and O_2SC, which appear to express that the higher the TLim-vVO_2max was, the higher the O_2SC amplitude was expected to be, being in accordance with other groups (e.g. Gaesser and Poole, 1996). The cause of the O_2SC appearance is still a matter of debate, seeming to be explained by the increased number of recruited motor units in heavy efforts. In this sense, this concept is still difficult to use in training prescription.

2.3. Anaerobic System

Nonetheless the importance of aerobic capacity in running, swimming, cycling and rowing performance, the anaerobic energy system is a significant contributor during short distances, namely those lasting less than 2 min (Gastin, 2001). However, quantitative assessments of anaerobic metabolism are difficult, since invasive measures (e.g. muscle biopsies, blood samples and magnetic resonance) are costly and unavailable in a field test setting, once it demands knowledgeable technicians and require a considerable amount of sophisticated equipment.

In middle and long distance running events, anaerobic performance is expressed differently accordingly to the dependence of each event from its energetic supporting system: it is clear that an 800 m runner will spend much more energy from anaerobic pathways than a Marathon runner. However, it is not easy to identify the exact contribution of each body energy systems. In Table 4, it is possible to observe some proposals in running.

Table 4. Percentage values attributed by different authors to the contribution of different energetic systems, in different running events

Authors	Anaerobic	Aerobic
800m		
Spencer e Gastin (2001)	34%	66%
Duffield et al. (2005a)	40%	60%
1500m		
Spencer e Gastin (2001)	16%	84%
Duffield et al. (2005b)	23%	77%
5000m		
Newsholme et al. (1992)	12.5%	87.5%
Marajo et al. (1994)	20%	80%
Half Marathon		
Newsholme et al. (1992)	0-3%	97-100%
Péronnet et Thibault (1989)	5-10%	90-95%

The observed differences for each event can be justified by different methodological and instrumental procedures, as well as by the athletes' level.

Considering this topic, we have been using a two-speed test (Mader et al., 1980) based in a distance in accordance with the competition event (600, 1200 or 2000 m respectively for 800, 1500 and 5000 m, and Half Marathon runners). The selected distance is performed at different intensities (80% for the first and higher than 95% for the second repetition), with a complete interval between them. Blood lactate samples are taken in each recovery min after each repetition until the maximum lactate value is obtained. With this test is possible to understand the increase of [La⁻] with velocity, to compare the slopes, to balance results of velocity associated to certain [La⁻] values and to understand how an athlete is progressing in the [La⁻]/velocity relationship (Figure 10).

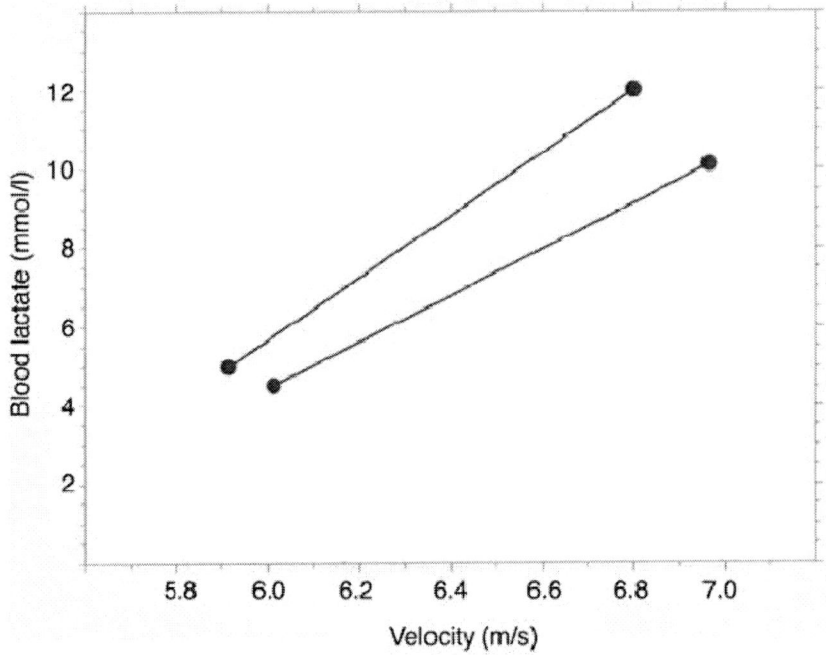

Figure 10. Graphical representation of two lines obtained from the two speed test, applied to a female runner (adapted from Colaço, 2007).

Thus, by using this test it is possible to compare the pattern of different lines obtained in different moments of the season, to better explain different competitive performance levels and to understand if the training process is promoting the expected levels of anaerobic adaptation. Simultaneously to the monitoring of the anaerobic changes, it should be observed the aerobic variations (through an AnT test) and have a better understanding of the relation between the test results and the specific performance changes for each event.

The purpose of our studieswere: (i) observing different performance levels between athletes (Colaço, 2007) and (ii) comparing the same athlete in different moments (Pedro, 2006). So, using the two-speed test, it was used the slope and area values trying to find the athlete with less increase [La⁻] rate with velocity increment, especially for intensities that are related with the athlete's event. In this perspective, we can notice that, for events with a significant anaerobic contribution, the lines patter at higher intensities can be more performance discriminative, particularly when aerobic level seems to be similar between athletes with different performance levels (Figure 11).

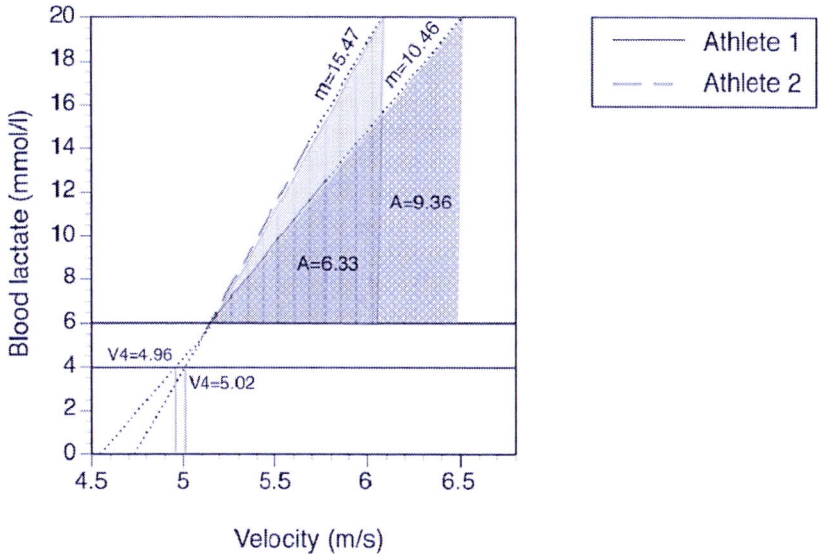

Figure 11. Representation of the two speed test of two 1500 m runners, with the slope (m) area obtained by the lines extrapolation until 20 mmol/l value and 6 m/s of running velocity (adapted from Colaço, 2007).

When this test is applied in middle distance runners, it is possible to observe different performance levels (Colaço, 2007). However, when we are working with 5000 m and Half Marathon runners, it seems that this test lose relevance. However, considering that some athletes can achieve similar aerobic levels, the specific use of some anaerobic contribution can determine different final results and also need to be taken in consideration in the training control and evaluation of these athletes. As an example, it is important to refer that the values obtained using the 2 x 2000 m test can be particularly discriminating of performance (Colaço, 2007), which happens particularly when the athletes with similar AnT have their performance level distinguished by the anaerobic energy contribution (Figure 12).

In swimming, knowing that the majority of the competitive events last less than 2 min, the importance of the anaerobic energy system is clearly stated. Holmér (1983) referred that for the 50 and 100 m events the anaerobic contribution is about 80%, or even more. Thus, a higher anaerobic capacity, with high rates of glycogen breakdown and glycolytic enzyme activities in the muscles, seem to be a prerequisite for fast swimming (Trappe, 1996). In this sense, in adittion to the traditionally used maximal [La⁻] values obtained in the final steps of incremental progressive tests or even in the end of short duration events, we have implemented some protocols to control and evaluate the anaerobic system contribution in swimming.

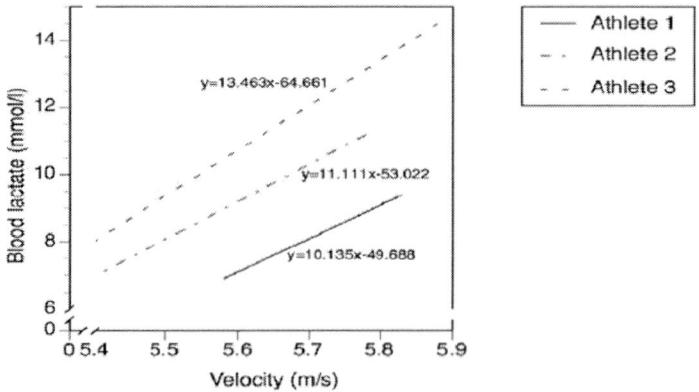

Figure 12. Lines and equations obtained throughout the two speed test for three 5000 m runners. Notice that the athlete 1 had the lower competitive level, although his higher anaerobic threshold (adapted from Colaço, 2007).

In a recent study, Fernandes et al. (2008a) proposed the anaerobic critical velocity test, assessed in front crawl, as a simple and non-invasive methodology that could allow coaches and scientists to have a new tool for swimmers training advice. This test was based on the concept of the (aerobic) critical velocity method, using the regression line equation obtained by the relationship between sprint distances and the respective time durations, to provide a hypothetical measure of the functional anaerobic capacity of swimmers. In Figure 13 it is possible to observe that anaerobic critical velocity was assessed through the slope of the regression equation established between the 12.5, 25 and 50 m test distances and the corresponding test times. Anaerobic critical velocity (represented as a and expressed in m/s) was calculated from the slope of the distance (y) versus time (x) relationship, and b is y-interception value, according to this equation:

$$y = ax + b \quad (1)$$

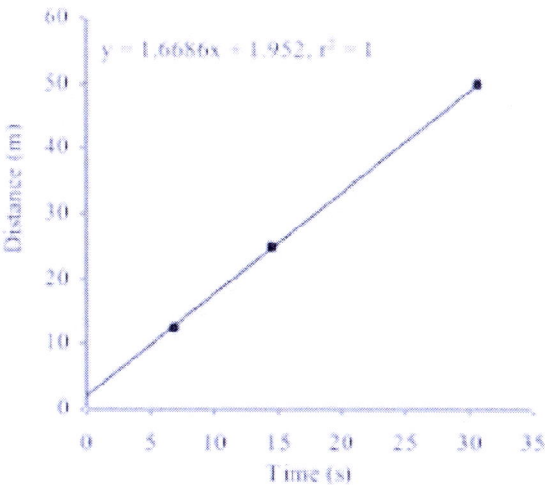

Figure 13. Example of a swimming anaerobic critical velocity assessment (Fernandes et al., unpublished data).

In the study of Fernandes et al. (2008a) it was found a strong inverse relationship between the anaerobic critical velocity and the 100 m front crawl time ($r = -0.84$), the first 50 m partial ($r = -0.87$) and the second 50 m partial ($r = -0.79$), all for a $p < 0.001$. Complementarily, the value of the anaerobic critical velocity converted in 100 m time was not different of the 100 m front crawl event duration. Even more recently, our group observed moderate to high correlation values between the anaerobic critical velocity and the specific velocities obtained in the 100 m butterfly, backstroke, breaststroke and freestyle events ($r > 0.60$, $p < 0.05$) (unpublished data). These authors also referred the absence of differences between anaerobic critical velocity and the velocity of the last 50 m of the above-referred events. Although future studies in larger samples should be advised, the preliminary results obtained suggest that anaerobic critical velocity can be used as measure of the anaerobic swimming potential.

Other area of interest, when referring to evaluating anaerobic swimming potential, is the assessment of fatigue thresholds. Nonetheless the study of fatigue thresholds is more evident at aerobic intensities, namely studying the AnT, we were able to observe the existence of velocity, force and power time-curves with one or two fatigue thresholds during 30 s tests (Soares et al., 2006 and Soares et al., 2008). Conducting five different tests with the same effort duration, being three general (cycloergometer Wingate test, crank ergometer Wingate test and simulated swimming on a biokinetic swim bench) and two specific (free swimming with connection to a cable velocimetric system and tethered swimming), it was observed that in the curves with one threshold, fatigue appears around 13 s from the beginning of the effort and, in curves with two fatigue thresholds, they become visible around 8 s and 18 s of exercise. In Figure 14, it is possible to observe a velocity-time trace of a swimmer in which the determined fatigue thresholds were plotted in (vertical lines).

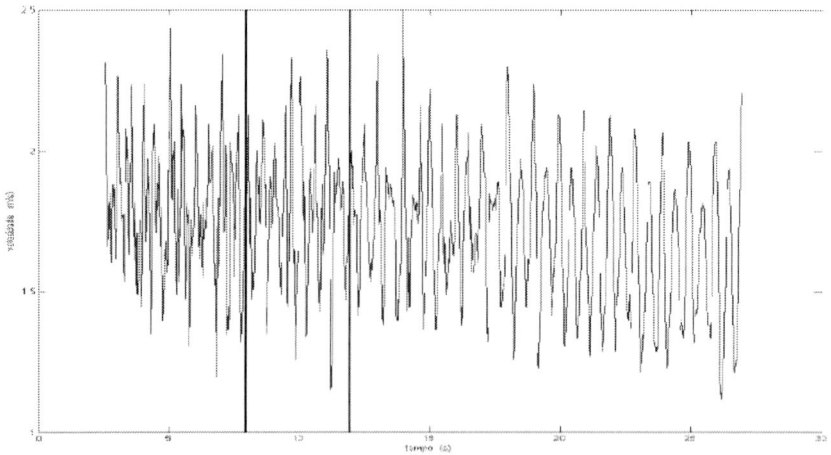

Figure 14. Velocimetric trace (with start, glide and arrival removed) of a swimmer with fatigue thresholds identified with vertical lines (Soares et al., unpublished data).

The above-referred authors concluded that fatigue thresholds appearance seem to be independent of the kind of effort performed by swimmers and speculate about the possibility of using velocity curves to determine an individual alactic-lactic threshold and better plan and control the anaerobic training. In this domain, the same authors have conducted a simple test for metabolic fatigue thresholds determination through [La$^-$] kinetics during an incremental 30 s protocol. Results showed differences in [La$^-$] near to 15 s swimming effort. Metabolic thresholds were close to velocimetric thresholds of v(t) curves.

3. CONCLUSION

We expect that the presented protocols, conducted in the bioenergetical area of expertise, could be well accepted and applied by athletes, coaches and scientists in their training control and athletes' evaluation programs. We keep on saying that reliable and systematic control and evaluation is a precious tool to increase the training efficiency and even contributing to predict performance.

As observed during the text, there is a large number of protocols to evaluate athletes and control the training process. Considering the different possibilities, we have been choosing those that allow getting the more applied results to training. Complementarily, we also have being trying to select tests with a good prediction capacity to help coaches and athletes to know the exact moments of the season to schedule their competitions.

One of our most important concerns has been to indirectly estimate some of the most used bioenergetical parameters and to state them in a comprehensible way to coaches and athletes. Finally, we expect to work in the future with as large number of athletes in longitudinal studies trying to perfect and individualize these methodologies.

REFERENCES

Bearden, S.E. and Moffatt, R.J. (2001). VO2 slow component: to model or not to model? *Med. Sci. Sports Exerc.*, 33 (4), 677-680.

Beneke, R. (1995). Anaeroboc threshold, individual threshold, and maximal steady state in rowing. *Med Sci Sports Exerc.*, 27 (6): 863-867.

Beneke, R. and von Duvillard, S. (1996). Determination of maximal lactate steady state response in selected sports events. Med Sci Sports Exerc, 28: 241-246.

Billat, V. (1998). *Physiologie et méthodologie de l'entraînement*. De la théorie à la pratique. De Boeck Université, Paris, France.

Billat, V.; Renoux, J.C.; Pinoteau, J.; Petit, B.; Koralsztein, J.P. (1994). Reproducibility of running time to exhaustion at VO2max in subelite runners. *Med. Sci. Sports Exerc.*, 2, 254-257.

Billat, V.; Faina, M.; Sardella, F.; Marini, C.; Fanton, F.; Lupo, S.; Faccini, P.; De Angelis, M.; Koralsztein, J.P.; Dal Monte, A. (1996). A comparison of time to exhaustion at VO2max in elite cyclists, kayac paddlers, swimmers and runners. *Ergonomics*, 39 (2), 267-277.

Billat, V.; Richard, R.; Binsse, V.M.; Koralsztein, J.P.; Haouzi, P. (1998). The VO2 slow component for severe exercise depends on type of exercise and is not correlated with time to fatigue. *J. Appl. Physiol.*, 85, 2118-2124.

Boiirgois J. and Vrijens J. (1998). Metabolic and cardiorespiratory responses in young oarsmen during prolonged exerci.se tests on a rowing ergometer at power outputs corresponding to two concepls of anaerobic threshold. *Eur J Appl. Physiol.*, 77: 164-9.

Canova R (2004). *Development of strenght endurance: the key to improve in middle and long distance events*. EACA Coaching Congress. Abano Terme. Italy.

Cardoso, C.; Fernandes, R.; Magalhães, J.; Santos, P.; Colaço, P.; Soares, S.; Carmo, C.; Barbosa, T.; Vilas-Boas, J.P. (2003). Comparison of a continuous and intermittent triangular protocols for direct VO2max assessment in swimming. In: J.-C. Chatard (edt.), *Proceedings of the IXth World Symposium on Biomechanics and Medicine in Swimming*, pp. 313-318. Saint-Etienne, France.

Cazorla, G. (1984). De l'evaluation en activité physique et sportive. Travaux et recherches en E.P.S. n° 7, *Evaluation de la valeur physique*, pp. 7-35. INSEP, Paris..

Colaço P (2007). Aerobic and anaerobic evaluation of middle distance and long distance runners (in Portuguese). Doctoral Thesis. Faculty of Sport, Porto University. Portugal.

Demarie, S.; Sardella, F.; Billat, V.; Magini, W.; Faina, M. (2001). The VO2 slow component in swimming. *Eur. J. Appl. Physiol.*, 84, 95-99.

Duffield R, Dawson B, Goodman C (2005). Energy contribution to 400-metre and 800-metre track running. *J. Sports Sci.*, 23 (3), 299-307.

Esteve-Lanao J., Juan A., Earnest C., Foster C., Lucia A. (2005). How do endurance runners actually trains? Relationship with competition performance. *Med. Sci. Sports Exerc.*, 37, 3: 496-504.

Fernandes, R. and Vilas-Boas, J.P. (1999). Critical velocity as a criterion for estimating aerobic training pace in juvenile swimmers. In: K. Keskinen, P. Komi, P. Hollander (eds.), *Proceedings of the VIII International Symposium of Biomechanics and Medicine in Swimming*, pp. 233-238. University of Jyvaskyla, Finland.

Fernandes, R.; Guerra, S.; Lamares, J.P.; Vilas-Boas, J.P. (2000). Critical velocity in swimming: three different methodologies for its determination. In: J. Avela, P. Komi and J. Komulainen (eds.), *Proceedings of the 5th Annual Congress of the European College of Sport Science*, pg 260. University of Jyvaskyla, Finland

Fernandes, R.; Billat, V.; Cardoso, C.; Barbosa, T.; Soares, S.; Ascensão, A.; Colaço, P.; Demarle, A.; Vilas-Boas, J.P. (2003a). Time limit at vVO2max and VO2max slow component in swimming. A pilot study in university students. In: J.-C. Chatard (edt.), *Proceedings of the IXth World Symposium on Biomechanics and Medicine in Swimming*, pp. 331-336. Saint-Etienne, France.

Fernandes, R.J.; Cardoso, C.S.; Soares, S.M.; Ascensão, A; Colaço, P.J.; Vilas-Boas, J.P. (2003b). Time limit and VO2 slow component at intensities corresponding to VO2max in swimmers. *Int. J. Sports Med.*, 24 (8): 576-581.

Fernandes, R.; Almeida, M.; Morais, P.; Machado, L.; Soares, S.; Ascensão, A.; Colaço, P.; Morouço, P.; Vilas-Boas, J.P. (2005a). Individual Anaerobic Threshold assessment in a swimming incremental test for VO2max evaluation. In: N. Dikic, S. Zivanic, S. Ostojic, Z. Tornjanski (eds.), *Abstract Book of the 10th Annual Congress of the European College of Sport Science*, pp. 266. Belgrade, Serbia.

Fernandes, R.J., Billat, V.L., Cruz, A.C., Colaço, P.J., Cardoso, C.S., Vilas-Boas, J.P. (2005b). Has gender any effect on the relationship between time limit at VO2max velocity and swimming economy? *J. Human Mov. Studies*, 49: 127-148.

Fernandes, R.J.; Billat, V.L.; Cruz, A.C.; Colaço, P.J.; Cardoso, C.S.; Vilas-Boas, J.P. (2006a). Does net energy cost of swimming affect time to exhaustion at the individual's maximal oxygen consumption velocity? *J. Sports Med. Phys. Fitness*, 46 (3): 373-80

Fernandes, R.; Cardoso, C.; Silva, J.; Vilar, S.; Colaço, P.; Barbosa, T.; Keskinen, K.L.; Vilas-Boas, J.P. (2006b). Assessment of time limit at lowest speed corresponding to maximal oxygen consumption in the four competitive swimming strokes. *Port. J. Sport Sci.*, 6 (2): 128-130.

Fernandes, R.J.; Aleixo, I..; Soares, S.; Vilas-Boas, J.P. (2008a). Anaerobic Critical Velocity: A New Tool for Young Swimmers Training Advice (chapter 10). In: N. P. Beaulieu (edt.), *Physical Activity and Children*: New Research, pp. 211-223. Nova Science Publishers, Inc. New York.

Fernandes, R.J., Keskinen, K.L., Colaço, P., Querido, A.J., Machado, L.J., Morais, P.A., Marinho, D.A., Vilas-Boas, J.P. (2008b). Time limit at VO2max velocity in elite crawl swimmers. *Int. J. Sports Med.*, 29: 145-150.

Gaesser, G.A. and Poole, D. (1996). The slow component of oxygen uptake kinetics in humans. *Exerc. Sport. Sci. Rev.*, 24.

Gastin, P.B. (2001). Energy system interaction and relative contribution during maximal exercise. *Sports Med.*, 31 (10), 725-41.

Heck, H.; Mader, A.; Hess, G.; Mucke, S.; Muller, R; Hollmann, W. (1985). Justification of the 4-mmol/l Lactate Threshold. *Int. J. Sports Med.*, 6: 117-130.

Holmér, I. (1983). Energetics and mechanical work in swimming. In A. P. Hollander; P. A. Huijing; G. de Groot (Eds.), Biomechanics and Medicine in Swimming (pp. 154-164). Campaign, Illinois: *Human Kinetics* Publishers.

Ingham, S.A.; Whyte, G.P.; Jones, K.; Nevill, A. (2002). Determinants of 2.000 m rowing ergometer performance in elite rowers. *Eur. J. Appl. Physiol.*; 88: 243-6.

Jones, A. and Doust, J. (1998). The validity of the lactate minimum test for determination of the maximal lactate steady state. *Med. Sci Sports Exerc*, 31: 1299-1306.

Jurimae, J.; Maestu, J.; Jiirimae, T. (2001). Blood laciale response to exercise and rowing pcrlbrmancc; relationships in competitive rowers. *J. Hum. Mov. Studies*, 41: 287-300

Koppo, K. and Bouckaert, J. (2002). The decrease in the VO2 slow component induced by prior exercise does not affect the time to exhaustion. Int. J. Sports Med., 23, 262-267.

Lucía, A.; Hoyos, J.; Chicharro, J.L. (2001). Physiology of professional road cycling. *Sports Medicine*, 31 (5): 325-337.

Mader, A.; Liesen, H.; Heck, H; Philippi, H.; Rost, R.; Schürch, P.; Hollmann, W. (1976). Zur Beurteilung der sportartspezifischen Ausdauerleistungsfähigkeit im Labor. *Sportarzt. Sportmed.*, 24 (4): 109.

Mader, A.; Madsen, O.; Hollmann, W. (1980). Zur beurteilung der laktaziden energiebereitstellung fur trainings-und wettkampfleistungen im schwimmen. *Leistungssport*, 10: 263-279.

Maestu, J.; Jurimae, J.; Jurimae, T. (2005). Monitoring of performance and training in rowing. *Sports Medicine*, 35 (7): 597-617.

Morais, P.; Almeida, M.; Aleixo, I.; Corredoura, S.; Colaço, P.; Machado, L.; Fernandes, R.; Vilas-Boas, J.P. (2006). Oxygen uptake at the lactate threshold in swimming. Port. *J. Sport Sci.*, 6 (2): 153-154.

Olbrecht, J. (2000). The science of winning. Planning, periodizing and optimizing swim training. *Swimshop*. Luton, England.

Olbrecht, J.; Madsen, O.; Mader, A.; Liesel, H.; Hullman, W. (1985). Relationship between swimming velocity and latic acid concentration during continuous and intermittent training exercise. *Int. J. Sports Med.*, 6 (2), 74-77.

Papadopoulos, C.; Doyle, J.; LaBudde, B.; Rupp, J.; Brandon, L.; Benardot, D.; Martin, D. (2003). Relationships between blood lactate parameters and endurance performance. *Med. Sci. Sports Exerc.*, 35 (5): 498.

Pedro, F. (2006). Aerobic evaluation of middle distance runners (in Portuguese). Masters Thesis. *Faculty of Sport, University of Porto. Portugal.*

Pyke, F. (2000). Introduction. In C. J. Gore (Edt.), Physiological tests for elite athletes (pp. xii-xiv). Australia: *Australian Sports Commission*.

Pyne, D.; Maw, G.; Goldsmith, W. (2000). Protocols for the physiological assessment of swimmers. In C. J. Gore (Edt.), Physiological tests for elite athletes, pp. 372-382. *Australian Sports Commission*. Australia.

Roecker, K; Schotte, O.; Niess, A.; Hortasmann, T.; Dickhuth, H. (1998). Predicting competition performance in long-distance running by means of a treadmill test. *Med. Sci. Sports Exerc.*, 30 (10): 1552-1557.

Santos P. and Ascencão A. (1999). Maximal lactate-steady-state in young male runners. International conference book. *"Youth Sports in the 21st Century", Michigan*.

Soares, S.; Fernandes, R.; Vilas-Boas, J.P. (2003). Analysis of critical velocity regression line informations for different ages: from infant to junior swimmers. In: J.-C. Chatard (edt.), *Proceedings of the IXth World Symposium on Biomechanics and Medicine in Swimming*, pp. 397-401. Saint-Etienne, France.

Soares, S.; Machado, L.; Lima, A.; Santos, I.; Fernandes, R.; Correia, M.; Maia, J.; Vilas-Boas, J.P. (2006). Velocimetric characterization of a 30 sec maximal test in swimming: consequences for bioenergetical evaluation. Port. *J. Sport Sci.*, 6: supl. 2,

Soares, S.; Aleixo, I.; Santos, I.; Machado, L.; Maia, J.; Vilas-Boas, J.P. (2008). Fatigue thresholds in 30s water and land exercises performed by swimmers. In: Cabri J, Alves F, Araújo D, Barreiros J, Dinis J, Veloso A (eds.), *Book of Abstracts of the 13th Annual Congress of the European College of Sport Science*, p. 500. Estoril, Portugal.

Spencer, M. and Gastin, P. (2001). Energy system contribution during 200 to 1500m running in highly trained athletes. *Med. Sci. Sports Exerc.*, 33 (1): 157-162.

Svedahl, K e MacIntosh, B. (2003). Anaerobic threshold: the concept and methods of measurement. *Can. J. Appl. Physiol.*, 28 (2): 299-323.

Trappe, S.W. (1996). Metabolic demands for swimming. In J.P. Troup; A.P. Hollander; D. Strasse; S.W. Trappe; J.M. Cappaert; T.A. Trappe (Eds.), *Biomechanics and Medicine in Swimming VII* (pp. 127-134). London: E & FN Spon.

Troup, J. (1995). *Physiological aspects of swimming*. Abstracts of the XI FINA World Sports Medicine Congress, pp. 65. FINA, Atenas.

Urhausen, A.; Coen, A. B.; Weiler, B.; Kindermann, W. (1993). Individual anaerobic threshold and maximum lactate steady state. *Int. J. Sports Med.*, 14 (3), 134-139.

Vilas-Boas, J.P.; Lamares, J.P:; Fernandes, R.; Duarte, J.A. (1997). Relationship between anaerobic threshold and swimming critical speed determined with competition times. *In: Abstract book of the FIMS's 9th European Congress of Sports Medicine. Porto, Portugal.*

Wakayoshi, K.; Ikuta, K.; Yoshida, T.; Udo, M.; Moritani, T.; Mutoh, Y.; Miyashita, M.; (1992). Determination and validity of critical velocity as an index of swimming performance in the competitive swimmer. *Eur. J. Appl. Physiol.* 64, 153-157.

Womack, C.J., Davis, S.E.; Wood, C.M.; Sauer, K.; Alvarez, J.; Weltman, A.; Gaesser, G.A. (1996). Effects of training on physiological correlates of rowing ergometry performance. *J. Strength Cond. Res.*, 10: 234-8

ACKNOWLEDGMENT

We thank José Bragada, from the Polytechnic Institute of Bragança (Portugal), for his review of this paper and for their pertinent suggestions.

In: Sports Medicine and Training Tools
Editors: B. Carmichael and A. Mitchell
ISBN: 978-1-61122-827-4
© 2011 Nova Science Publishers, Inc.

Chapter VI

BIOMECHANICS OF MARTIAL ARTS AND COMBATIVE SPORTS

Osmar Pinto Neto[*]

Texas A&M University, Texas, United States of America
Universidade Camilo Castelo Branco, Brazil
Instituto de Pesquisa e Qualidade Acadêmica (IPQA), Brazil

ABSTRACT

The pioneer studies on the biomechanics of martial arts were published in the nineteen sixties and seventies. After these articles were published, several other biomechanical studies have been conducted about martial arts and other related punching sports using a variety of different measures and methods, especially in the last decade. In general, these studies were concerned with the enhancement of performance and extending the understanding of injury risk. This paper presents a comprehensive review on this subject. It is divided in two major topics: the first topic covers articles about the kinetics, kinematics and electromyography of specific hand strikes, kicks, throws and fall techniques; the second topic focus on some aspects of motor behaviors and perceptual abilities fundamental for efficient and successful performances in martial arts and combative sports (i.e. repeatability of movement, reaction times).

---

[*] e-mail osmarpintoneto@hotmail.com

1. Introduction

In the past 15 to 20 years the participation of athletes in martial arts and combative sports has increased dramatically (Oler et al., 1991; Pieter and Lufting, 1994). Along with the increase in participation an increase in the number of scientific papers published about martial arts and combative sports has also increased. These manuscript reviews the advancements made on the biomechanics of martial arts and combative sports.

Fights among unarmed men are probably as old as men themselves, in contrast scientific studies of fighting are very recent. The pioneer studies on this subject were published in the 1960s and 1970s. Vos and Binkhorst (1966) were fundamental to set start the scientific investigations of martial arts with their article entitled "Velocity and force of some karate arm-movements" published at "Nature". During the 1960s, other important article was published, entitled "Karate strikes", by J.D. Walker (1975) in the American Journal of Physics. Finally, in 1978 an article entitled "The physics of karate" by Feld, McNair and Wilk published in the Scientific American, would contribute largely to the popularization of the studies on the biomechanics of martial arts.

After these articles were published, several other biomechanical studies have been conducted about martial arts and other related punching sports using a variety of different measures and methods, especially in the last decade. In general, these studies were concerned with the enhancement of performance and extending the understanding of injury risk. This paper presents the first review on this subject. It is divided in two major topics: the first topic covers articles about the kinetics, kinematics and electromyography of specific hand strikes, kicks, throws and fall techniques; the second topic focus on some aspects of motor behaviors and perceptual abilities fundamental for efficient and successful performances in martial arts and combative sports (i.e. repeatability of movement, reaction times).

1.1 Different Styles of Martial Arts and Combative Sports

The articles cited in this review are based on results coming from five different modalities: Kung Fu, Karate, Taekwondo, Judo and Boxing. This section gives a brief description of these styles.

1.1.1 Kung Fu

Kung fu is a popular term that expresses Chinese martial arts in general. Colloquially, the term "kung fu" in Chinese alludes to any individual accomplishment or cultivated skill obtained by long and hard work. The origins of Kung Fu can be traced over 6,000 years ago to self-defense needs, hunting activities and military training in ancient China. From this beginning, Chinese martial arts proceeded to incorporate different philosophies and ideas into its practice expanding its purpose from self-defense to health maintenance and finally as method of self-cultivation. Through Chinese kung fu history, various warriors developed different techniques (styles) of self-defense with particular sets of movements and ideas (Despeux, 1981). Most of these styles were developed as progressions and offshoots of the styles created in two main ancient schools of martial arts in China (Reid & Croucher, 1983). These schools were located at two philosophical and religious centers, the Shaolin Temple (Buddhist) and the Wudang Mount (Taoist) (Despeux, 1981). Today there are more hundreds of Kung Fu styles. Although its popularity, the great number of styles and its ancient history, studies on the biomechanics of Kung Fu are still rare.

1.1.2 Karate

Karate is one of the most widespread martial art and combative sport; it involves primarily the use of punches, kicks and blocking techniques (Halabchi et al., 2007). There are not nearly as much styles of Karate as there is of Kung Fu; the main differences among Karate styles are in the way they compute, since their strikes, punches and kicks are similar. Due to its early wide popularity in the United States Karate was the first martial art to be investigated scientifically (Vos and Binkhorst, 1966).

Karate began as a common fighting system known as "te" among the samurai class of the Ryukyu Islands. Riukyu Islands are located west of China between Japan and Taiwan; Okinawa is its largest island. Still in its early history, two main factors furthered the development of karate in Okinawa. The first, in 1372, was the establishment of trade relationships between Okinawa and the Ming dynasty of China, which caused many forms of Chinese martial arts to be introduced to Okinawa. The second was the 'Policy of Banning Weapons,' enforced in Okinawa during the late 1400's. (Reid and Croucher, 1983)

Because of the Chinese influence, the word karate was originally a way of expressing "Chinese hand." In 1933, the Okinawan art of karate was recognized as a Japanese martial art and karate started to be written in Japanese characters now as "empty hand". (Higaonna, 1985)

1.1.3 Taekwondo

Taekwondo is a Korean martial art very popular worldwide and the national sport of South Korea. In Korean, tae means "foot"; kwon means "fist"; and do means "way". Traditional Taekwondo is typically not competition-oriented and stems from military roots. Modern Taekwondo, which is much more popular, on the other hand, tends to emphasize competition. Formally, there are two main styles of Taekwondo. Although there are doctrinal and technical differences between the two main styles and among the various organizations, the art in general emphasizes kicks. The roots of Taekwondo go back thousands of years. In 1955, a number of similar schools of martial arts were merged, and the resulting style was named Taekwondo. An important figure in this effort was Choi Hong Hi, a Korean general who worked to combine a traditional Korean foot-fighting technique called "tae kyon" with Japanese Karate. In 1966, General Choi established the International Taekwondo Federation (ITF) (Tae Kwon Do, 2008). As for Kung Fu, studies on the biomechanics of Taekwondo are also rare.

1.1.4 Judo

Judo is a modern Japanese martial art and combat sport that originated in Japan in the late nineteenth century. Unlike Kung-fu, Karate and Taekwondo there is only one style of Judo. Its most prominent feature is its competitive element, where the ultimate goal is to either throw one's opponent to the ground at his back, or immobilize or force one's opponent to quit with grappling maneuvers. Judo was developed by Jigoro Kano (1860–1938). In 1880, Kano reformed an ancient Japanese martial art called jujutsu with a new set of rules for competition and with focus on development of the body, mind and character of the practitioners. The word "judo" is formed by two characters: "ju", which means soft method and "do", which means, as in Taekwondo, way, road or path. (Group, 1977)

1.1.5 Boxing

Boxing, also known as Western boxing or pugilism, is a combat sport in which two participants, generally of similar weight, fight each other with their fists wearing padded gloves. Boxing is supervised by a referee and is typically engaged in during a series of one to three-minute rounds. Victory in boxing can be achieved in three different ways: by points at the end of the bout, given by judges' scorecards; by Knockout, when a fighter is knocked down and unable to get up before the referee counts to ten seconds; or by Technical Knockout, when a fighter is considered too injured to continue. (Group, 1977)

Boxing first appeared as a formal Olympic event in the 23rd Olympiad (688 BC), but fist-fighting contests must certainly have had their origin in mankind's prehistory. The earliest visual evidence for boxing appears in Sumerian relief carvings from the 3rd millennium BC (boxing, 2008). Modern boxing evolved in Europe, particularly Great Britain. During the early 18th century, in Great Britain, boxing was done bare-knuckle and referred to as prizefighting. The first documented account of a bare-knuckle fight in England appeared in 1681 in the London Protestant Mercury. This is also the time when the word "boxing" first came to be used (Roberts and Skutt, 1999). Pugilism is a much older word, it indicates the ancient origins of the sport in its derivation from the Latin "pugil", which mean a boxer, related to the Latin "pugnus", which means fist, and derived in turn from the Greek "pyx", which means with clenched fist (boxing, 2008).

2. KINETICS, KINEMATICS AND ELECTROMYOGRAPHY OF MARTIAL ARTS AND COMBATIVE SPORTS

Since the beginning of martial arts biomechanics research, scientists were intrigued in quantifying the forces involved in strikes performed by highly trained subjects. Recently, although still in a discrete manner, a few articles have been published trying to understand how trained subjects can achieve such performances. Along with that, there have been a few attempts to compare trained and untrained subjects' performances. These studies are important not only for the enhancement of performance but the understanding of injury risk. Recently, advancements have been made in the quantification of the forces that are exerted on the human body, when hit by a martial arts or combative sport strike during a real fight or competition. Other advancement recently made in the biomechanics of martial arts relates to the quantification of ground reaction forces during fall. Research indicates that martial arts techniques present ways to reduce forces exerted in the human body during falls. This topic covers articles about the kinetics, kinematics and electromyography of specific hand strikes, kicks, throws and fall techniques.

2.1 Biomechanics of Hand Strikes and Kicks

2.1.1 Kinetics and Kinematics

Joch et al. (1981) measured average punch impact forces of 3453 N for elite and 2932 N for intermediate boxers. Wilk et al. (1983) reported that adept karate practitioners could obtain maximum speeds values in the range of 5.7-9.8 m/s when performing straight punches, and impact forces in the range of 2400-2800 N when hitting a concrete patio block. Voigt (1989) built a dynamometer to analyze punches of 10 well trained karate students. He found peak impact force of 3334 N (2345 - 4866 N), and maximal speed of the hand before impact of 9.5 m/sec (8.2 - 10.7 m/s). Smith et al. (2000) measured average impact forces, using a sport-specific designed dynamometer, of 4800 N (SD = 601) for elite and 3722 N (SD = 375) for intermediate boxers. Gulledge (2008) compared mechanical factors in the reverse and three-inch power punches performed by twelve expert male Karate martial artists. They used a force plate to measure horizontal peak forces, and subsequently impulses. The power punch produced smaller fist velocities immediately before impact than the reverse punch, 4.09 vs. 6.43 m/s. The peak force exerted by the fist was much smaller in the power punch than in the reverse punch 790 vs. 1450N. However, they found that the linear impulse exerted by the fist during the first 0.20s of contact was slightly larger in the power punch than in the reverse punch (43.2 vs. 37.7N.s). They concluded that the power punch is less powerful than the reverse punch, but slightly more effective for throwing the opponent off balance.

The values of force shown above were not estimated considering impacts to objects comparable in mass and biofidelity to segments of the human body, thus the risk of injury cannot be reliably estimated from these forces. In an effort to better understand the relationship between forces delivered to human body and the risk of injury, a few studies have been conducted. Schwartz et al (1986) investigated the relative force of kicks and punches thrown at a dummy head, which was mounted 175 cm above the floor, their mechanism was contrived to provide constant rotational stiffness, and springs provided constant restorative moments about the three axes. They asked fourteen karate experts to punch and kick the dummy and measured accelerations ranging from 90 to 120 g. Walilko et al. (2005) submitted Olympic class boxers to perform straight punches thrown at an instrumented Hybrid III headform that simulated a human head. They calculated impact force and impact power values for seven boxers' punches and obtained an average impact force of 3427 N (SD = 811) and an average impact power of 6574 W (SD = 3453); they reported an average hand speed of 9.14 m/s (SD = 2.06). Pierce et al., (2006) obtained the first direct measurement of punch force in professional boxing matches through boxing gloves incorporating the *bestshot* System ™, a proprietary system created by SensorPad Systems, Inc. (SPS; Norristown, PA). They obtained force data across all rounds of six professional boxing matches across five different weight classes. Mean punch forces delivered ranged from 866.6 N to 1149.2 N. These measurements are considerably less than those reported above found in laboratory demonstrations, and may better reflect the actual forces exchanged in the ring. More studies should be done in order to verify if these forces do represent better the forces exchanged during actual boxing matches.

Several articles have made contribution in the attempt to understand how martial artists could obtain such values of force and power as described above, and why and how they perform different than untrained subjects. Wilk et al. (1983) suggested that the hand speed right before the impact was the primary factor contributing for the greater impact force of a karate martial artist strike compared to a non-martial artist. However, they did not verify this suggestion in their study. Walker (1975) suggested that another important variable, the effective mass of impact, could vary in different forms of karate strikes and affect the impact force; however, he did not report values of this variable.

The effective mass of impact is a measure of a body's inertial contribution to the transfer of momentum during a collision. In the case of a martial art strike, the effective mass can be seen as the mass of an imaginary rigid body that could replace the striker and with the same speed as the hand speed before the impact produce the same effect on the collision as the striker would. Blum (1977) suggested that an adept Karate practitioner achieves a "high mass" by tightening all the appropriate arm and upper body muscles at the moment of impact, but further insight into this theory was not provided.

Smith and Hamill (1986) were the first authors to investigate this suggestion. They measured the fist velocities from karate athletes of different skill levels and the relative momentum of a 33 kg punching bag. The bag momentum was greatest for the highest skilled subjects compared to the lower skilled punchers even though their respective fist velocities were approximately the same (11.03 (standard deviation (SD) 1.96) m/s for all subjects). Smith and Hamill (1986) suggested that the increase in bag momentum was due to the skilled boxer's ability to generate a greater effective mass during the impact than the lower skilled boxers. The estimated average effective mass for the highest skilled boxers was approximately 4.1 kg. Since this value is greater than the mass of the hand, the authors believed it reflected the ability of the athletes to link the mass of the arm into the punch. Voigt (1989) found the effective mass of karate punches calculated from calibrated punching dynamometer to be 1.4 kg (1.0 - 2.2 kg) and calculated from stroboscopic recordings to be 4.0 kg (2.5 - 4.5 kg). Walilko et al. (2005) reported a mean effective punch mass of 2.9 (SD 2.0) kg and a slight linear association of the effective mass with the weight of the boxer.

Neto et al. (2007c) was the first study that calculated values of effective mass from both trained and untrained subjects. In their study, the subjects were asked to strike a basketball at rest on a table five times with maximum force using a palm strike. Kung Fu athletes presented significantly higher averages of effective mass, hand speed and performance (ball speed after collision) than control group. The average effective mass for the Kung Fu group was 2.62 (SD 0.33) kg and for the control group was 1.33 (SD 0.19) kg. The average hand speed was 6.67 (SD 1.42) m/s for the Kung Fu group and 5.04 (SD 0.57) m/s for the control group. The average ball speed was 9.00 (1.89) m/s and 5.72 (SD 0.44) m/s for the Kung Fu group and control group, respectively. Comparing the values obtained for the average effective mass and hand and forearm mass estimated using regression equations, the authors found that for the control group the effective mass was statistically equivalent to the mass of the hand and forearm, while for the Kung Fu group the effective mass was significant greater than the mass of the hand and forearm. Contrary to what was found by Walilko et al. (2005), for both groups and all subjects no significant correlation was found between the values of effective mass and body mass. The authors concluded that because of the higher effective masses of the KF athletes, the KF group performance increases approximately twice as much with the increase of hand speed than the performance of the control group and that the effective mass is the main factor that distinguish a trained from a non-trained subject. Accordingly, Neto et al. (2008b) found a significant linear relationship between the values of average muscle and impact power for experienced Kung Fu Yau-Man practitioners, but not for the non-experienced participants. In other words, for the experienced participants an increase in muscle power was directly reflected in an increase in impact power, while for the non-experienced participants a higher muscle power did not necessarily corresponded to a higher impact power.

There are not as many studies on the biomechanics of kicks as there is of hand strikes. All articles reviewed are based on kicks performed by taekwondo athletes. Pieter and Pieter (1995) measured forces up to 620 N for the round kick against a water-filled bag with a built-in force sensor unit. Conkel, et al. (1988) used piezoelectric film, similar to that used to measure pressure distribution on the foot during gait, and attached it to a heavy bag to measure the impact force of front, side, back and roundhouse kicks. Impact forces of up to 470 N were recorded for the roundhouse kicks. Pieter and Pieter (1995), Conkel, et al. (1988) and Serina and Lieu (1991) have measured linear velocity of the foot immediately before impact during the execution of the round kick ranging from 14 to 16 m/s. Boey et al. (2002) reported kinematical results of turning kick performance of 4 athletes, two men and two women, in the Singapore National Taekwondo squad. Kicks speeds ranged from 11.53 to 15.04 m/s for the women and 17.12 to 22.7 m/s for the men. Pedzich et al. (2006) investigated the side-kick and spinning back kick performed by 5 competitors with mastery class of taekwondo. They reported average maximal stroke force values of 9015±2382 N (right leg) and 8294±2308 N (left leg) for the side-kick and 8569±2381 N (right leg) and 7751±2570 N (left leg) for the spinning back kick. Tsai et al. (2007) reported values of ankle speed of 9.55±1.65 m/s for the spin-whip kick performed by eight elite Taekwondo male college students.

2.1.2 Electromyography

As far as I know only three articles on the electromyography of hand strikes were published. Neto et al. (2007a) compared the electromyographic activity of the triceps brachii, biceps brachii and brachioradialis muscles during palm strikes with and without impacts. Electromyography analyses were done in the time and wavelet domains. Morlet wavelet power spectra were obtained and an original method was used to quantify statistically significant regions on the power spectra. The results both in the time and frequency domains indicated higher triceps brachii and brachioradialis muscle activity for the strikes with impacts. No significant difference was found for the biceps brachii in the two different scenarios. Neto et al. (2008a) reported a kinematical and electromyographic analysis of Kung Fu Yau-Man Palm strikes without impact. An empirical model applied to data obtained by a high-speed camera (1000 Hz) described the kinematical characteristics of the movement. Similar to Neto et al. (2007a), the authors analyzed the electromyographic patterns of the biceps brachii, brachioradialis and triceps brachii muscles during the strike in the time and frequency domains. The electromyography results showed a well developed muscle coordination of the practitioners in agreement with kinematical results. In an attempt to further understand the difference between highly trained martial arts athletes and untrained subjects, Neto et al. (2007b) evaluated the coordination between agonists and antagonists muscles of the arm in a movement of Kung Fu performed by trained and untrained subjects. The authors demonstrated, using wavelet transforms to analyze the data in the frequency domain through time, that the untrained subjects presented much higher undesired co-contractions during the strikes.

Electromyographic studies of kicks are also very rare. Sorensen et al. (1996) examined whether proximal segment deceleration during kicks is performed actively by antagonist muscles or is a passive consequence of distal segment movement, and whether distal segment acceleration is enhanced by proximal segment deceleration. Their results were based on data collected from seventeen skilled taekwondo practitioners were filmed using a high-speed camera while performing a high front kick, and electromyography recordings from five major lower extremity muscles. Their results indicated that thigh deceleration was caused by motion-dependent moments arising from lower leg motion and not by active deceleration.

Aggeloussis et al. (2007) conducted a research to study the repeatability of electromyography waveforms of major lower limb muscles during the axe kick in taekwondo. They recorded data from the rectus femoris, biceps femoris, gastrocnemius lateralis and tibialis anterior during 10 successive kicks performed to a fixed target by each participant. The electromyographic activity during the kicks presented coefficient of variation greater than 80%. The authors concluded that only ensemble averages of electromyography waveforms obtained from more than ten kicks may be considered representatives of the muscle function in this type of kicks.

2.2 Throws and Falls

To date, only a handful of studies have investigated judo from a biomechanical perspective. Harter and Bates (1985) studied the ground reaction forces associated with the harai-goshi throw. A tri-modal peak anteroposterior ground reaction forces pattern indicating a pull-push-pull effort by thrower was found during the throw. Tezuka et al. (1983) also measured the ground reaction forces of haraigoshi and found similar results.

Pucsok et al., (2001) analyzed and compared the kinetic and kinematic characteristics of the throwing technique Harai-goshi (hip throw), of novice and advanced judo competitors. Kinetic and kinematic data were collected by utilizing the Kistler Instrument Corporation Multicomponent Force Measuring Platform System and the Peak Technologies Motion Video Analysis System. This article revealed a significant difference in horizontal force application, between novice and advanced judo competitors. Numerous significant relationships among mean horizontal ground reaction force application and horizontal leg sweep velocity in was found in 19 of the 28 participants of the study. They suggested that leg sweep velocity is a function of ground reaction force application and horizontal leg sweep velocity plays a primary role in good technical execution of the Harai-goshi throw.

Imamura and Johnson (2003) recorded twenty male judo players, 10 black belts and 10 novices, executing the major outer leg reap with maximal effort. Statistical analysis found that peak angular velocity of the trunk and peak angular velocity of the ankle differed significantly from the performance of the experienced and novice participants. These differences were attributed to good upper body to upper body contact or impact, and stressed the importance of executing plantar flexion near sweep contact. Their results emphasized the importance of using the sweeping leg in a sequential kinetic link motion rather than as a single rigid segment.

Imamura et al. (2006) filmed and analyzed four black belt throwers in three dimensions using two video cameras (JVC 60 Hz) and motion analysis software. They investigated three different throwing techniques: Harai-goshi (hip throw), Seoi-nage (hand throw), and Osoto-gari (leg throw). Each throw was broken down into three main phases; balance breaking, fit-in and actual throw. Their results showed that for the Harai-goshi and Osoto-gari throws, impulse measurements were the largest within the first two phases of the movement. The Seoi-nage throw demonstrated the lowest impulse and maintained forward momentum on the body of faller throughout the entire throw.

Imamura et al. (2007) was the first article to consider the biomechanics of judo throwing out of isolated laboratory conditions. They compared the kinematics of throwing under competitive and non-competitive conditions under a real-life competitive condition and a simulated laboratory condition. Their results were based on data collected from a third degree black belt subject served as the thrower for both conditions, and two black belt participants ranked as first degree and fourth degree that served as the faller. They found that the directional velocity patterns of the peak velocity for the center of mass of the thrower and faller were similar in both conditions. They did find differences in timing and magnitude of peak center of mass directional velocity and peak angular velocity of the thrower's trunk. During competition, thrower created larger peak center of mass directional velocities onto the faller, which indicated greater throwing power. Peak velocities for thrower center of mass were larger during the noncompetitive condition since faller resistance was minimal.

As much as martial arts practitioners train to throw opponents to the ground, they must train to fall to the ground without getting hurt. For that, martial artists train specific fall techniques. For almost a decade, it has been suggested that that martial arts fall techniques can reduce hip impact forces (Sabick et al., 1999). Groen et al. (2007) quantified the role of hand impact, impact velocity, and trunk orientation in the reduction of hip impact force in martial arts techniques. In their study six experienced judokas performed sideways falls from kneeling height using three fall techniques: using the arm to break the fall, martial art rolling technique with use of the arm to break the fall, and martial art technique without use of the arm. Their results showed that the martial art technique can reduced the impact force by approximately 30%. Impact velocity was also significantly reduced in the falls done with the rolling technique. They found no significant differences between the rolling techniques using and without using the hands. The fact martial arts fall technique can contribute to the reduction of impact forces without using the arm to break the fall provided support for the incorporation of these techniques in fall prevention programs for elderly. Weerdesteyn et al. (2008) took one step further and investigated whether hip impact forces and velocities in martial arts falls would be smaller than simply using the arm to break the fall in ten young adults without any prior experience after a thirty minutes training session in sideways martial arts fall techniques. They found that martial arts falls had significantly smaller hip impact forces (17%) and velocities (7%). They concluded that training in martial arts techniques is very promising with respect to their use in interventions to prevent fall injuries.

3. Motor Behaviors and Perceptual Ability

Successful performance in martial arts and combative sports requires efficient execution of motor behavior and a high level of perceptual ability. This topic reviews articles about a couple of fundamental aspects of motor behavior and perceptual ability, repeatability of movement and reaction time.

3.1 Repeatability of Movement

The quantitative analysis of the repeatability of martial arts strikes and combative sports can help the better understanding of practitioners' motor control, as well as serve as a valuable tool for training. Ravier and Millot (1999) analyzed links between decision-making and motor control through karate techniques. In their study six karate practitioners had to perform two movements previously automatized in three experimental situations. The first was a simple situation in which the subject had no opponent and had to perform the parries (only one possibility). The second was a situation with choice, in which the subject still had no opponent and had to perform one of the parries at the trainer's request (two possibilities). In the third situation the subjects had to choose between the two movements to lock the attack of an opponent. They measured angular variations of elbow and knee joints as well as their duration were measured, using goniometry and showed a significant decrease in the precision of technical skills in the third situation compared with the simple situation.

Sforza et al. (2000) quantified the repeatability of the displacement of thirteen body landmarks of seven karate practitioners while performing two different basic karate hand strikes. Subjects were filmed with an optoelectronic computerized instrument (100 Hz) while performing 10 repetitions of straight punches and lunge punches. From the data of each subject, they calculated the average time of execution and the standard deviations of each of the three spatial coordinates x, y, z were computed for each landmark. The results showed that for all subjects, the execution of lunge punch took longer. For both punches and almost all landmarks, the largest repeatability (smallest standard deviation) was found in the vertical direction, while the smallest was found in the anteroposterior direction (direction of movement). Considering all karate practitioners, they showed that the lunge punch had a total standard deviation about 3 to 6 times larger than that measured during the performance of straight punches. In a similar study, Sforza et al. (2002) studied the repeatability of the karate front kick when performed by 13 black belt karate practitioners. The results showed that two experienced athletes presented the lower variability. The best repeatability was found in the horizontal plane, and in general for the hips and head movements.

Roosen and Pain (2007) examined the execution of a popular kicking combination during training in two level of intensity. 3D movement data were captured at 250Hz using a VICON motion analysis system from five taekwondo practitioners. They found that execution in two different intensity levels cause changes in angle data. Their data suggested that the first kick in the sequence showed the most differences in general. For all kicks, most differences are seen in the central segments. Angles related to the head and to the pelvis show most variability.

3.2 Reaction Time

In sport science, two types of perceptual abilities have been considered relevant to player's successful performance. One is primitive, basic sensory functions which are not specific to particular types of sport expertise. The other type of perceptual processing is sport-specific perceptual skills (Mori, 2002). Research on the perceptual abilities of martial artists and combative sports athletes is scarce. Layton (1993), citing one of his previous studies (Layton,

1991), reported that reaction time for hitting a punch bag in response to a sound stimulus were faster for karate black belts, although the reaction times of the advanced athletes did not differ in proportion to their grades. Kim and Petrakis (1998) the administered Identical Pictures Test, a time-constrained multiple-item test of perceptual judgments, to 50 male and 45 female volunteer karate practitioners who were classified by skill and belt-rank into three groups. Their results showed that black belts and the women had faster visual-perceptual speed.

Lee et al., (1999) reported that the reaction time to perform a ballistic finger extension movement in was significantly shorter in kendo (143 +/- 12 ms) and karate (146 +/- 11 ms) athletes compared to sedentary subjects (176 +/- 12 ms). They suggested that the RT is shortened through motor learning in the kendo and karate athletes who trained for momentary movements. Williams and Elliott (1999) have used more realistic stimuli and tasks to examine expertise anticipation of karate athletes, which is one important aspect of perceptual skill. In their study, the stimuli were dynamic film displays of karate athletes performing offensive attacks against the viewer. The film was presented on a large screen to give a real-size view of the performing athletes. The participant's task was a choice reaction time task, where the participants had to respond differently, as soon and accurately as possible, to the attacking positions. In this scenario, anticipating the attacking position from an early part of the video sequence would lead to faster reaction times and/or higher accuracy. The results showed that expert karate athletes were no faster but more accurate than the novices. In a similar study Mori et al. (2002) investigated simple reaction times, choice reaction times and anticipation of karate athletes. Their results showed significant differences between the karate athletes and the novices in the choice reaction time task, but not in the simple reaction time. O'Donovan et al. (2006) examined simple reaction times, choice reaction times and movement times of thirteen Taekwondo and Kung Fu practitioners and a control group. The experiment consisted of the subjects releasing an initiation button and depressing a stop button 25 cm away. Results indicated that during the simple and choice reaction time tasks the martial artists were no quicker in lifting their hand off a button in response to a sound stimulus, but were significantly faster in moving to press another button. Fontani et al. (2006) examined 18 karate practitioners, 9 of High Experience and 9 of Low Experience and showed that experience Karate practitioners reacted faster than those of low experience on the simple RT test (204 vs. 237 ms, $p < .01$).

Perez (2006) presented an extensive study on reaction time of karate athletes. In his study, 169 adults practitioners of karate, and 32 non-practitioners performed a choice reaction time test created using a computer software called SuperLab Pro version 2.0 (Cedrus Corporation, USA). Reaction time task consisted on pushing a button of a computer keyboard as quickly as possible, when a black square appeared on the screen. The black square could be in four different positions, and the subject had to press a different key according with the position. Each subject performed the test one hundred times and the authors calculated their efficiency in the task considering the reaction time and the number of mistakes made. They also collected personal and sport data using a questionnaire, tapping test in 10, 20 and 30 seconds data and hand grip strength data. Comparisons were made considering the subjects' competition specialty (fighting or forms), sport rank (regional, national without medal, national with medal and international) and sex. No significant differences were found in any of the comparisons. They also found that karate athletes were no different than the general population in the choice reaction time task. They found that reaction time was correlated to tapping and hand grip strength. They also found differences in reaction time depending on gender, concluding that men were faster than women.

4. FINAL REMARK

This manuscript has presented a comprehensive review on the biomechanics of martial arts and combative sports. It has described the advancements made in this area, especially in the topics of kinetics, kinematics, electromyography and perceptual and motor skills. Most of the studies available in the literature are related to hand strikes, kicks, throws and fall techniques from five different modalities: Kung Fu, Karate, Taekwondo, Judo and Boxing.

REFERENCES

Aggeloussis, N., Vassilis, G., Sertsou, M., Giannakou, E. & Mavromatis, G. (2007). Repeatability of electromyographic waveforms during the Naeryo Chagi in taekwondo. *Journal of Sports Science and Medicine, 6(CSSI-2)*, 6-9.

Blum, H. (1977). Physics and the art of kicking and punching. *American Journal of Physics, 45*, 61-64.

Boey, L.W. & Xie, W. (2002). Experimental investigation of turning kick performance of Singapore national Taekwondo players. Proceeding of ISBS, Caceres – Spain, 302-305. boxing. (2008). In Encyclopaedia Britannica,

2008/12/12, Available from: Encyclopædia Britannica Online: *http://www.bri tannica.com/EBchecked/topic/76377/boxing*

Chow, D. & Spangler, R. (1982). *Kung Fu, History, Philosophy and Technique.* North Hollywood, CA: Unique Publications

Conkel, B. S., Braucht, J., Wilson, W., Pieter, W., Taaffe, D., & Fleck, S.J. (1988). Isokinetic torque, kick velocity and force in taekwondo. *Medicine and Science in Sports and Exercise, 20(2),* S5.

Despeux, C. (1981). *Tai-Chi Chuan: Arte Marcial Técnica de Longa Vida* (5th edition). São Paulo, SP: Círculo do Livro S.A. (in Portuguese).

Feld, M. S., McNair, R. E., & Wilk, S. R. (1979) The physics of karate. *Scientific American, 240(4),* 150-158.

Fontani, G., Lodi, L., Felici, A., Migliorini, S. & Corradeschi, F. (2006) Attention in athletes of high and low experience engaged in different open skill sports. *Perceptual & Motor Skills. 102(3),* 791-805.

Groen, B.E., Weerdesteyn, V. & Duysensa, J. (2007) Martial arts fall techniques decrease the impact forces at the hip during sideways falling. *Journal of Biomechanics, 40,* 458–462.

Group, D. (1977). Enjoying Combat Sports. (1st edition) New York, NY, Paddington Press.

Gulledge, J.K. & Dapena, J. (2008). A comparison of the reverse and power punches in oriental martial arts more options. *Journal of Sports Sciences, 26(2),* 189-196

Halabchi, F., Ziaee, V. & Lotfian, S. Injury profile in women Shotokan Karate Championships in Iran (2004-2005) (2007) *Journal of Sports Science and Medicine 6(CSSI-2),* 52-57.

Harter, R.A. & Bates, B.T. (1985). Kinematic and temporal characteristics of selected judo hip throws. Proceedings of ISBS, Del Mar, CA, 141-150.

Higaonna, *M.* (1985). *Traditional Karatedo-1 Fundamental Techniques.* Tokyo: Minato Research and Publishing Co. Ltd.

Imamura. R. & Johnson, B. (2003) A kinematic analysis of a judo leg sweep: major outer leg reap-osoto-gari. *Sports Biomech*anics, *2(2),* 191-201.

Imamura, R. T., Hreljac, A., Escamilla, R. F. & Edwards, W. B. (2006). A three-dimensional analysis of the center of mass for three different judo throwing techniques. Journal of Sports Science and Medicine, 5 (CSSI), 122 – 131.

Imamura, R. T., Iteya, M., Hreljac, A. & Escamilla, R. F. (2007) A kinematic comparison of the judo throw Harai-goshi during competitive and non-competitive conditions. Journal of Sports Science and Medicine, 6(CSSI-2), 15-22.

Joch, W., Fritche, P., & Krause, I. (1981). Biomechanical analysis of boxing. In K. Morecki, K. Fidelius, K. Kdzior & A. Wit (Eds.), Biomechanics VII-A (343-349). Baltimore, MD: University Park Press.

Kim, H.S. & Petrakis, E. (1998). Visuoperceptual speed of karate practitioners at three levels of skill. *Perceptual & Motor Skills, 87(1)*, 96-98.

Layton, C. (1991). How fast are the punches and kicks of traditional Shotokan karateka? *Traditional Karate, 4*, 29–31.

Layton, C. (1993) Reaction time + movement-time and sidedness in Shotokan karate students. *Perceptual & Motor Skills, 76*, 765-766.

Lee, J.B., Matsumoto, T., Othman, T., Yamauchi, M., Taimura, A., Kaneda, E., Ohwatari, N. & Kosaka, M. (1999). Coactivation of the flexor muscles as a synergist with the extensors during ballistic finger extension movement in trained kendo and karate athletes. *International Journal of Sports Medicine 20*, 7-11.

Mori, S., Ohtani, Y. & Imanaka, K. (2002). Reaction times and anticipatory skills of karate athletes. *Human Movement Science* 21, 213-230.

Neto, O. P., Magini, M., & Pacheco, M. T. T. (2007a) Electromyographic study of a sequence of Yau-Man Kung Fu palm strikes with and without impact. *Journal of Sports Science and Medicine, 6, 23-27.*

Neto, O.P., Magini, M., Marzullo, A. C. M. & Pacheco, M.T.T. (2007b). Estudo Eletromiográfico da coordenação entre músculos agonistas e antagonistas do braço durante um golpe de Kung Fu Yau-Man. *Terapia Manual, 4*, 303-306. (In Portuguese)

Neto, O. P., Magini, M., & Saba, M. M. F. (2007c) The role of effective mass and hand speed in the performance of kung fu athletes compared to non-practitioners. *Journal of Applied Biomechanics, 23*, 139-148.

Neto, O. P., & Magini, M. (2008a) Electromyography and kinematic characteristics of Kung Fu Yau-Man palm strike. *Journal of Electromyography and Kinesiology, 18*, 1047-1052.

Neto, O.P., Magini, M., Saba, M. M. F. & Pacheco, M.T.T. (2008b) Comparison of Force, Power, and Striking Efficiency for a Kung Fu Strike Performed by Novice and Experienced Practitioners: Preliminary Analysis. *Perceptual and Motor Skills, 106*, 188-196.

O'Donovan, O., Cheung, J., Catley, M., McGregor, A. H. & Strutton, P. H. (2006). An investigation of leg and trunk strength and reaction times of hard-style martial arts practitioners. *Journal of Sports Science and Medicine, CSSI*, 5-12.

Oler, M., Tomson, W., Pepe, H., Yoon, D., Branoff, R. & Branch, J. (1991) Morbidity and mortality in the martial arts: a warning. *The Journal of Trauma, 31,* 251–253.

Pedzich, W., Mastalerz, A. & Urbanik, C. (2006). The comparison of the dynamics of selected leg strokes in taekwondo WTF. *ACTA of Bioengineering and Biomechanics, 8,* 63-81.

Pérez, O.M.Q. (2003). El tiempo de reacción visual en el Karate. PhD. thesis - Universidad Politécnica de Madrid. (In Spanish).

Pierce, J. D. Jr., Reinbold, K. A. Lyngard, B. C., Goldman, R. J. & Pastore, C.M. (2006) Direct Measurement of Punch Force During Six Professional Boxing Matches, Journal of Quantitative Analysis in Sports [http://www.bepress.com/jqas/vol2/iss2/3] 2(2).

Pieter, F., & Pieter, W. (1995). Speed and force in selected taekwondo techniques. *Biology of Sport, 12(4),* 257-266.

Pieter, W. & Lufting, R. (1994) Injuries at the 1991 taekwondo world championships. *Journal of Sports Traumatology and Related Research, 16,* 49–57.

Pucsok, J.M., Nelson, K., Ng ED. (2001) A kinetic and kinematic analysis of the Harai-goshi judo technique. *ACTA Physiologica Hungarica, 88 (3-4),* 271-280.

Rasch, P. J., & Pierson, W. R. (1963). Reaction and movement time of experienced karateka. *The Research Quarterly, 34,* 242–243.

Ravier, G. & Millot, J. L. (1999). Etude des ajustements moteurs mis en oeuvredans des situations d'apprentissage (kihon) et appliqués en karate. *Science & Sports, 14,* 130-136 (in French).

Reid, H., & Croucher, M. (1983). *The way of the warrior: the paradox of the martial arts.* (2nd edition) London: Century Pub.

Roberts, J.B. & Skutt, A.G. (2002). *The Boxing Register* (3rd edition) Ithaca, NY McBooks Press.

Roosen, A. & Pain, M. T. G. (2007). Kinematic changes in the reproduction of a taekwondo kicking combination. *Journal of Biomechanics, 40,* 455-455.

Sabick, M.B., Hay, J.G., Goel, V.K. & Banks, S.A. (1999). Active responses decrease impact forces at the hip and shoulder in falls to the side. *Journal of Biomechanics 32,* 993–998.

Schwartz, M.L., Hudson, A.R., Fernie, G.R., Hayashi, K. & Coleclough, A. A. (1986) Biomechanical study of full-contact karate contrasted with boxing. *Journal of Neurosurgery, 64(2),* 248-252.

Serina, E.R., Lieu, D.K. (1992) Thoracic injury potential of basic competition taekwondo kicks. *Journal of Biomechanics, 25(10),* 1247-8.

Sforza, C., Turci, M., Grassi, G., Fragnito, N., Pizzini, G. & Ferrario, V.F. (2000) The repeatability of choku-tsuki and oi-tsuki in traditional Shotokan karate: a morphological three-dimensional analysis. *Perceptual & Motor Skills, 90(3 Pt 1),* 947-60.

Sforza, C., Turci, M., Grassi, G.P., Shiray, Y.F., Pizzini, G. & Ferrario, V.F. (2002) Repeateability of Mae-Geri_Keage in tradiotional Karate: A three-dimensional analysis with black-belt karateka. *Perceptual & Motor Skills, 95,* 433-444.

Smith, M. S., Dyson, R. J., Hale, T. & Janaway, L. (2000) Development of a boxing dynamometer and its punch force discrimination efficacy. *Journal of Sports Sciences, 18*, 445-450.

Smith, P.K. & Hamill, J. (1986). The effect of punching glove type and skill level on momentum transfer. *Journal of Human Movement Studies 112,* 153-161.

Sorensen, H., Zacho, M., Simonsen, E., Dyhre-Poulsen, P. & Klausen, K. (1996) Dynamics of the martial arts high front kick. *Journal of Sports Sciences, 14*, 483-495.

Tae Kwon Do. (2008). In Microsoft Encarta Online Encyclopedia, 2008/12/12, Available from: http://encarta.msn.com/encyclopedia_761585873/Tae_Kwon_Do.html

Takahashi, R. (1992). The application of biomechanics to judo technique "OKURI-ASHI-BARAI" (Sweeping Ankle Throw). *Sports coach, 15,* 30-33.

Tezuka, M., Funk, S., Purcell, M. & Adrian, M. (1983). Kinetic Analysis of judo technique. In: *Biomechanics, VIII-B*. Eds: Matsui, H. & Kobayashi, K. Champaign, IL: Human Kinetics. 869-875.

Voigt, M. (1989). A telescoping effect of the human hand and forearm during high energy impacts t. *Journal of Biomechanics, 22(10),* 1065.

Vos, J. A. & Binkhorst, R. A. (1966). Velocity and force of some Karate arm-movements. *Nature, 211*, 89-90.

Walilko, T. J., Viano, D.C. & Bir, C.A. (2005). Biomechanics of the head for Olympic boxer punches to the face. *British Journal of Sports Medicine, 39,* 710-719.

Walker, J. D. (1975). Karate Strikes. *American Journal of Physics, 43*, 845-849.

Weerdesteyn, V., Groen, B. E., Van Swigchem, R. & Duysens, J. (2008) Martial arts fall techniques reduce hip impact forces in naïve subjects after a brief period of training. *Journal of Electromyography and Kinesiology, 18,* 235–242.

Wilk, S.R., McNair, R. E. & Feld, M. S. (1983). The Physics of Karate. *American Journal of Physics, 51*, 783-790.

Williams, A. M. & Elliott, D. (1999). Anxiety, expertise, and visual search strategy in karate. *Journal of Sport & Exercise Psychology, 21*, 362–375.

Reviewed by Prof. Marcio Magini, PhD. Universidade Camilo Castelo Branco and Instituto de Pesquisa e Qualidade Acadêmica (IPQA), Sao Paulo – Brazil.

INDEX

A

abuse, 36
activity level, vii, viii, 40, 42, 43, 44, 45, 49, 52, 53, 55, 58
adaptation, 70, 78
adaptations, 72
administration, 13
administrators, 32, 33
adolescents, 23, 42, 43, 55, 56, 57
adult obesity, 40
adulthood, 33, 52
adults, 100, 102
aerobic, ix, 62, 64, 65, 74, 76, 78, 79, 80, 81, 84
aerobic capacity, 65, 76
age, 4, 63, 65, 66, 67
aggression, 29, 31, 37
anabolic steroids, 22, 30, 35
anaerobic, ix, 62, 64, 65, 66, 70, 72, 76, 77, 78, 79, 80, 81, 82, 83, 84, 87
angular velocity, 99
antagonists, 97, 98
Anxiety, 108
application, 98, 107
assessment, vii, ix, 46, 57, 58, 59, 61, 64, 68, 81, 84, 85, 87
Australia, 86, 87
availability, 63

B

basketball, 12, 13, 19, 96
behaviors, x, 12, 19, 42, 89, 90
biceps brachii, 97
biceps femoris, 98
biomechanics, vii, ix, 89, 90, 91, 92, 93, 96, 99, 103, 107
blood, ix, 62, 65, 66, 68, 69, 70, 71, 72, 74, 75, 76, 86
body size, viii, 39, 44, 47, 49, 52, 53
boxer, 93, 96, 107
brachioradialis, 97
Brazil, 89, 108
breakdown, 29, 80
breaststroke, 81

C

capacity, ix, 62, 64, 65, 76, 80, 83
capillary, 66, 75
case study, vii, 2, 3, 4, 7
causality, 42
causation, 43
CBS, 35
Census, 41, 59
CFI, ix, 40, 49, 51
chemotherapy, 9
childhood, viii, 39, 40, 41
China, 35, 91
class, 91, 94, 97

clinical assessment, 58
coaches, ix, 2, 4, 6, 7, 8, 13, 14, 16, 61, 62, 63, 64, 65, 66, 70, 75, 80, 82, 83
coding, viii, 11, 13
coefficient of variation, 98
cognitive activity, 46, 47
cognitive dissonance, 57
cognitive theory, viii, 39, 40, 42, 54, 56
college students, 97
colleges, 22
collisions, 6
communication systems, 34
competition, vii, 2, 3, 5, 6, 11, 12, 13, 14, 16, 17, 18, 24, 25, 32, 33, 34, 62, 63, 66, 67, 74, 75, 77, 84, 87, 88, 92, 93, 99, 103, 106
competitive conditions, 99, 104
competitive sport, 9
competitor, 4
competitors, 97, 98
compliance, 35
components, 4
computer software, 102
concentration, 65, 68, 70, 73, 74, 86
concrete, 94
conditioning, 5
conference, 8, 87
confidentiality, 28
Congress, 84, 85, 87, 88
consent, 24, 35, 47
constitutionality, 26
constraints, 66, 75
consumption, 68, 85
contractions, 97
control, ix, 9, 61, 62, 63, 64, 67, 73, 79, 80, 82, 83, 96, 100, 102
control group, 96, 102
coronary heart disease, 41
correlation, 28, 29, 46, 49, 66, 72, 81, 96
correlation coefficient, 28
correlations, 46, 49
cost, 24, 41, 85
costs, 12
CP, 73, 74
criticism, 31
cultivation, 91

cultural, 18
cultural influence, 18
culture, viii, 11, 12, 16, 17, 18, 19
cycling, ix, 61, 62, 63, 64, 65, 69, 76, 86
cyclists, 69, 83

D

data analysis, 13
data collection, 54
defense, 91
degree, 5, 16, 17
demographic, viii, 11, 13
demonstrations, 95
Department of Health and Human Services, 56, 58
desire, 13, 14, 16
detection, 31, 32
diagnosis, 7, 9, 62
direct measure, 94
directors, viii, 21, 27, 28, 29, 31, 33, 34, 36
discomfort, 44
discrimination, 107
diseases, 4, 9
displacement, 101
drug testing, 24, 26, 27, 31, 32, 35, 36, 37
drugs, 12, 19, 22, 23, 27, 30, 31, 32, 33, 34, 35, 36
dry, 6
duration, 69, 75, 80, 81, 101

E

Education, 19
educational process, 33
electromyography, x, 64, 89, 90, 93, 97, 98, 103
elementary school, 53
employment, 54
encouragement, 44, 52, 53, 54
endurance, vii, 75, 84, 86
energy, ix, 62, 64, 65, 70, 76, 77, 79, 85, 107
England, 8, 34, 86, 93
English, 16, 18
environment, vii, 11, 12, 66
epidemic, viii, 39, 41

Index

epidemiology, 7
evolution, 63, 72
execution, 97, 98, 100, 101
Executive Order, 24
exercise, vii, 62, 65, 69, 72, 73, 74, 76, 82, 83, 85, 86
experiences, 17, 18, 57
expert, 94, 102
expertise, 82, 101, 102, 108
exposure, 42
extrapolation, 79

F

facilitators, 54
factor analysis, 46
fatigue, 2, 81, 82, 83
film, 96, 102
Finland, 84
flexor, 105
focusing, 64, 74
football, 4, 6, 12, 24, 25, 30, 55
foundations, 56
Fourth Amendment, 26
France, 83, 84, 87
frequencies, 4

G

gait, 96
gastrocnemius, 98
gender, 12, 13, 14, 17, 18, 66, 85, 103
gender differences, 12, 13, 14, 17, 18
gloves, 92, 95
grades, 24, 35, 102
Great Britain, 93
groups, 5, 76, 96, 102
guardian, 24, 25
guidance, 54
guidelines, vii, 1, 6, 7, 51, 69
gymnastics, 47

H

health, 12, 18, 91
health care costs, 41

health care system, 41
heart, 69, 74
Heart, 69
heart disease, 41
herpes, vii, 1, 2, 3, 4, 5, 6, 7, 8, 9
herpes labialis, 4
herpes simplex, 2, 3, 8, 9
herpes simplex virus type 1, 8, 9
high school, vii, viii, 1, 2, 3, 4, 7, 22, 23, 24, 25, 26, 27, 28, 30, 31, 32, 33, 34, 36, 37, 40, 43, 45, 53, 55
high-speed, 97, 98
hip, 98, 99, 104, 106, 107
hospitalization, 2
human, 93, 94, 107
Human Kinetics, 19, 85, 107
hypertension, 41
hypothesis, 17

I

identification, 63
Illinois, 85
image, 14, 16, 47
impacts, 94, 97, 107
implementation, vii, 1
independence, 13
individualization, 68
infection, 2, 3, 4, 9
infections, 8
infectious, 3, 6
initiation, 102
injuries, 5, 6, 11, 12, 100
injury, vii, x, 2, 6, 11, 12, 13, 16, 17, 18, 19, 63, 89, 90, 93, 94, 106
insight, 5, 95
intensity, 69, 76, 101
intercollegiate athletics, 3, 26
nterpersonal relationships, 17
interval, 66, 73, 77
invasive, 76
Iran, 104
Ireland, 41, 57
Islam, 46, 58
island, 91
ISS, 12

Italy, 84

J

Japan, 91, 92
Japanese, 91, 92
joints, 101

K

kindergarten, viii, 39, 44, 47
kinematics, x, 64, 89, 90, 93, 99, 103
kinetics, x, 74, 76, 82, 85, 89, 90, 93, 103

L

lead, 2, 70, 102
learning, 40, 43, 102
legality, 26, 30
legislation, 24, 32
leisure, viii, 39, 42, 46, 49
leisure time, viii, 39, 49
likelihood, vii, 1, 3, 4, 6, 7
limitations, 17, 65
Limitations, 34, 54
linear, 69, 94, 96
London, 87, 93, 106
long distance, 65, 66, 67, 77, 84
longitudinal studies, 83
longitudinal study, 42
Louisiana, 23

M

magnetic resonance, 76
Maine, 2, 8
maintenance, 75, 91
majority, viii, 16, 29, 31, 33, 39, 41, 45, 48, 49, 53, 54, 65, 79
management, vii, 2, 3, 4, 6, 7, 8
measurement, 76, 87, 94
measures, ix, 76, 89, 90
media, 22, 30, 54
median, 46
medicine, 7, 8, 19
membership, 18
men, 12, 16, 17, 18, 90, 97, 103

Mercury, 93
metabolic, 65, 69, 76, 82
metabolic rate, 76
metabolism, 76
methodological procedures, 74
methodology, 67, 80
Microsoft, 107
military, 91, 92
Ming dynasty, 91
modalities, ix, 61, 62, 63, 64, 90, 103
modality, 63, 76
modeling, 41, 43, 53, 54, 58
momentum, 95, 99, 107
monitoring, 78
morphological, 107
mortality, 106
motion, 98, 99, 101
motivation, 16
motives, 17, 18
motor behavior, x, 89, 90, 100
motor control, 100
motor skills, 103
movement, x, 64, 89, 90, 97, 98, 99, 100, 101, 102, 105, 106
multiples, 45
multivariate statistics, 59
muscle, 76, 96, 97, 98
muscle mass, 24
muscle power, 96
muscles, 80, 95, 97, 98, 105

N

national, vii, 1, 92, 103
National Collegiate Athletic Association, 3, 8, 12, 18
National Collegiate Athletic Association (NCAA), 12
NCAA, 7, 8, 12
negotiation, 19
New England, 8, 34
New York, 85, 104
Nixon, 12, 16, 18
non-invasive, 66, 80
norms, viii, 11, 12, 17

O

obesity, viii, 39, 40, 41, 42, 44, 56, 57, 58, 59
observational learning, 40, 43
observed behavior, 42
opportunities, 3, 29, 34, 43, 54
optoelectronic, 101
organization, 5
organizations, 6, 7, 92
overtraining, 63
overweight, 41, 56, 58
overweight adults, 41
oxygen, ix, 62, 68, 74, 76, 85
oxygen consumption, 68, 85

P

pain, vii, 11, 12, 13, 14, 16, 17, 18, 19, 27, 32
paper, x, 64, 88, 89, 90
paradox, 106
parameter estimates, 52
parental influence, 54, 59
parental support, 43
parenting, 43, 57
parents, 14, 16
Paris, 83, 84
passive, 98
path analysis, 48, 49
path model, 42, 44, 49, 52
pathways, 70, 77
peer influence, 56
perceptual judgments, 102
perceptual processing, 101
performance, iv, vii, ix, x, 22, 23, 24, 30, 31, 32, 33, 34, 35, 61, 62, 63, 64, 66, 68, 75, 76, 77, 78, 79, 83, 84, 86, 87, 88, 89, 90, 93, 96, 97, 99, 100, 101, 103, 105
performance-enhancing substances, 23, 32, 34
permission, iv, 47
permit, 33
personal, 6, 103
philosophical, 91
phosphates, 65
physical activity, vii, viii, 40, 41, 42, 43, 44, 45, 46, 49, 52, 53, 54, 55, 56, 57, 58, 59

physicians, 6, 7
physics, 90, 104
physiological, ix, 62, 64, 65, 67, 70, 87, 88
physiological correlates, 88
physiology, 62
piezoelectric, 96
plantar flexion, 99
play, vii, 11, 12, 13, 14, 16, 18
population, 2, 103
Portugal, 61, 84, 86, 87, 88
positive relation, 76
positive relationship, 76
power, ix, 62, 64, 68, 74, 81, 83, 94, 95, 96, 97, 99, 104
precedent, 5
pre-competitive, 72
prediction, 63, 83
preparation, 5
pressure, 16, 96
prevention, 32, 63, 100
prior knowledge, 31
procedures, 5
promote, 72
protection, 2
protocol, 67, 69, 74, 82
protocols, 62, 64, 65, 69, 80, 82, 83, 84
proximal, 97
psychology, iv
punishment, 25

Q

questionnaire, viii, 11, 13, 103

R

race, 18, 30
reaction time, x, 27, 89, 90, 100, 102, 105
recall, 42, 59
recreational, 19, 74, 76
recruiting, 70
rectilinear, 68
rectus femoris, 98
reduction, 99
regional, 103
regression, 80, 87, 96

Index

regression equation, 80, 96
regression line, 80, 87
relationship, 12, 13, 17, 78, 80, 81, 85, 94, 96
relationships, 67, 76, 86, 91, 98
relevance, 67, 79
reliability, 13, 28, 46, 56, 57
repeatability, x, 89, 90, 98, 100, 101, 107
repetitions, 101
reproduction, 40, 42, 106
research, 12, 16, 17, 62, 93, 98
researchers, viii, 11, 13
risk, vii, viii, x, 1, 2, 3, 4, 6, 7, 8, 11, 12, 16, 18, 19, 89, 90, 93, 94
risk management, vii, 1, 3, 4, 6, 7, 8
risks, 3, 6, 16, 18
rolling, 100
rowing, ix, 61, 62, 63, 64, 65, 68, 76, 83, 86, 88
rugby, 3, 9
rumination, 17

S

safety, 2, 18
schizophrenia, 57
scholarship, 5, 22, 33
school, vii, 1, 2, 3, 4, 5, 7, 91, 92
school activities, 34, 46
scientific knowledge, vii
scientists, ix, 62, 64, 65, 66, 80, 82, 93
SCT, 53
sedentary behavior, 46, 47, 56
sedentary lifestyle, 41, 52
self-efficacy, 43, 54
self-presentation, viii, 11
self-regulation, 54, 56
Senate, 25
Serbia, 85
series, 65, 75, 92
sex, 103
shoulder, 2, 106
signals, 51
signs, 33
Singapore, 97, 103
skills, 5, 101, 103, 105
skin, 2, 4, 5, 6, 7, 8

social, 8
social construct, 8
socialization, 57
society, 5, 17, 18
socioeconomic status, 53, 54
software, 99, 102
South Korea, 92
Spain, 103
spatial, 101
specialists, 63
specificity, 68, 69, 76
spectrum, 63
speed, 67, 68, 77, 78, 79, 80, 85, 87, 94, 95, 96, 97, 98, 102, 105
spin, 97
sports, viii, ix, 4, 7, 8, 11, 13, 18, 61, 62, 63, 64, 68, 75, 83, 89, 90, 100, 101, 103, 104
SPSS, 13
standard deviation, 48, 49, 95, 101
Statistical Package for the Social Sciences, 13
steroids, vii, viii, 21, 22, 23, 24, 25, 27, 28, 29, 30, 31, 32, 33, 34, 35
stiffness, 94
stimulus, 102
strain, 3
strains, 6
strength, 103, 105
strikes, x, 89, 90, 91, 93, 95, 96, 97, 100, 101, 103, 105
stroke, 41, 97
strokes, 75, 85, 106
structural equation modeling, 58
students, 2, 84, 94, 97, 105
substance use, 38
suicide, 22
summer, 4
Supreme Court, 26, 27, 30, 33
surveillance, 35
survey, 28, 30, 34, 35
swimmers, 67, 74, 75, 76, 80, 82, 83, 84, 85, 87
symptoms, vii, 1, 2, 3, 7, 29, 31, 33
systems, ix, 62, 64, 65, 77

T

Taiwan, 91
talent, 22
team sports, 62
technicians, 77
testing, 23, 24, 25, 26, 27, 30, 31, 32, 33, 34, 35, 36, 37, 38, 63, 69, 72
testing program, 24, 25, 26, 32, 35, 36, 63
testosterone, 34, 37
test-retest reliability, 46
three-dimensional, 64, 104, 107
threshold, ix, 62, 65, 66, 69, 72, 80, 82, 83, 86, 87
thresholds, 81, 82, 87
tibialis anterior, 98
time, vii, 1, 4, 68, 74, 80, 81, 83, 85, 86, 93, 97, 101, 102, 105, 106
training, iv, vii, ix, 17, 22, 32, 61, 62, 63, 64, 65, 67, 69, 70, 72, 73, 75, 76, 78, 79, 80, 82, 83, 84, 86, 88, 91, 100, 101, 107
transcript, 3, 8
transcripts, 36
transfer, 95, 107
transformation, 48
transmission, 4, 5, 58

U

United States, 91
university students, 84
unreasonable searches, 26, 33

V

validation, 55, 58, 59
validity, 86, 88
valuation, 62, 84
values, 12, 17, 65, 66, 67, 68, 69, 73, 74, 75, 76, 77, 78, 79, 80, 81, 94, 95, 96, 97
variability, 63, 68, 75, 101
variable, 95
variations, 78, 101
velocity, ix, 62, 65, 66, 67, 68, 69, 70, 71, 72, 73, 74, 78, 79, 80, 81, 82, 84, 85, 86, 87, 88, 96, 98, 99, 104
video, 47, 49, 99, 102
video games, 47, 49
videos, 47
virus, 2, 3, 8
virus infection, 8
viruses, 2, 9
visible, 82
visual, 2
VO, 74, 75, 76

W

wages, 53
walking, 45, 46, 48, 52
water, 62, 87, 96
wavelet, 97
weight loss, 2
White House, 32, 38
WHO, 9
wind, 62
winning, 5, 14, 86
women, 12, 16, 17, 18, 97, 102, 103, 104
World Health Organization, 2, 9

Y

young adults, 100